Instructor's Manual to Accompany

3-2-1 Code It!

Second Edition

Michelle A. Green, MPS, RHIA,
FAHIMA, CMA (AAMA), CPC, PCS
SUNY Distinguished Teaching Professor
Department of Physical & Life Sciences,
Alfred State College, Alfred, NY

Contributing Authors
Sarah Serling, CPC, CPC-H, CPC-I, CCS, CCS-P, CCS
Clinical/Technical Editor, Ingenix, Eden Prairie, MN

Lynette Williamson, MBA, RHIA, CCS, CPC
Instructor, Health Information Technology
Santa Barbara City College, Santa Barbara, CA

DELMAR
CENGAGE Learning

Australia • Brazil • Japan • Korea • Mexico • Singapore • Spain • United Kingdom • United States

DELMAR
CENGAGE Learning

**Instructor's Manual to Accompany
3-2-1 Code It! Second Edition**
Michelle A. Green and Lynette Williamson

Vice President, Career and Professional Editorial: Dave Garza

Director of Learning Solutions: Matthew Kane

Senior Acquisitions Editor: Rhonda Dearborn

Managing Editor: Marah Bellegarde

Product Manager: Jadin Babin-Kavanaugh

Editorial Assistant: Chiara Astriab

Vice President, Career and Professional Marketing: Jennifer McAvey

Executive Marketing Manager: Wendy Mapstone

Senior Marketing Manager: Nancy Bradshaw

Marketing Coordinator: Erica Ropitzky

Production Director: Carolyn Miller

Production Manager: Andrew Crouth

Senior Content Project Manager: James Zayicek

Senior Art Director: Jack Pendleton

Technology Project Manager: Ben Knapp

For product information and technology assistance, contact us at
Professional & Career Group Customer Support, 1-800-648-7450

For permission to use material from this text or product,
submit all requests online at **www.cengage.com/permissions.**
Further permissions questions can be e-mailed to
permissionrequest@cengage.com

2009 Current Procedural Terminology © 2008 American Medical Association. All rights reserved.

Library of Congress Control Number: 2008929261

ISBN-13: 978-1-4354-4828-5

ISBN-10: 1-4354-4828-6

Delmar
5 Maxwell Drive
Clifton Park, NY 12065-2919
USA

Cengage Learning products are represented in Canada by Nelson Education, Ltd.

For your lifelong learning solutions, visit **www.delmar.cengage.com**

Visit our corporate website at **www.cengage.com**

Printed in the United States of America
1 2 3 4 5 XX 11 10 09

Contents

Preface

This Instructor's Manual is organized into seven sections:

- Section I: Preparing Your Course
- Section II: Answer Keys to Chapter Exercises and Reviews
- Section III: Chapter Exams and Answer Keys to Chapter Exams
- Section IV: Answer Keys to Workbook Assignments and Reviews
- Section V: Answer Keys to Workbook Appendices A-D: Coding Patient Records
  - Answer Key to Appendix A: Coding Ambulatory Care Surgery Patient Records
  - Answer Key to Appendix B: Coding Emergency Department Patient Records
  - Answer Key to Appendix C: Coding Physician Office Records
  - Answer Key to Appendix D: Coding Hospital Inpatient Records
- Section VI: Answer Key to Workbook Appendix E: Mock Certified Professional Coder (CPC) Certification Examination
- Section VII: Answer Key to Workbook Appendix F: Mock Certification Coding Specialist-Physician (CCS-P) Certification Examination (available at Online Companion)

Section I (Preparing Your Course) assists instructors in the organization of the course. Sample semester plans are provided along with policies for administering exams and grading assignments and exams. The purpose of creating lesson plans is discussed, and chapter lesson plans that can be modified for individual use are included. Section II (Answer Keys to Chapter Exercises and Reviews), Section III (Chapter Exams and Answer Keys to Chapter Exams), and Section IV (Answer Keys to Workbook Assignments and Reviews) are organized according to chapter. Detailed feedback is located below answers to clarify assigned codes. Section V (Answer Keys to Workbook Appendices A-D: Coding Patient Records) is organized according to patient case number, and detailed feedback is included below answers to clarify assigned codes. Section VI (Answer Key to Workbook Appendix E: Mock Certified Professional Coder (CPC) Certification Examination) and Section VII (Answer Key to Workbook Appendix F: Mock Certification Coding Specialist Physician (CCS-P) Certification Examination) contains answers to the mock exams.

> **Note:**
>
> *Chapter exams (and answers) in this Instructor's Manual contain questions that are different from those found in the computerized test bank in the Instructor's Resource. The chapter exams are the same as those included in the WebTutor™, which provides detailed feedback for the answers.*

> **Teaching Tip:**
>
> *For ease of reference in locating the sections in the Instructor's Manual, consider placing a sticky note as a tab at the beginning of each section.*

STUDYWARE

The StudyWare CD-ROM located inside the back cover of the textbook allows students to review concepts learned in each chapter and to assign codes to practice cases.

> ### Teaching Tip:
>
> *StudyWare is an automated study guide for students. Instead of publishing (and selling!) a separate study guide of questions for students to complete, Cengage Delmar Learning bundles StudyWare with the textbook. Your students will notice that all types of questions are included in StudyWare (e.g., multiple choice, matching, true/false, fill-in-the-blank, and "open" coding). The software organizes the questions in a game format (e.g., fill-in-the-blank as hangman and crossword puzzles), which makes it fun for students to use.*

ENCODER PRO

The Encoder Pro CD-ROM located inside the back cover of the textbook contains Ingenix's powerful medical coding solution that allows you to look up ICD-9-CM, CPT, and HCPCS Level II codes quickly and accurately. This software can be used to assign codes to any of the exercises in the *3-2-1 Code It!* textbook and work-book. (Be sure to check with your instructor before installing the Encoder Pro software because the CD-ROM bundled with your book expires 30 days after installation.)

ONLINE COMPANION

Additional resources can be found online at **http://www.delmarlearning.com/companions**. Click on 'Allied Health' from the left navigation menu, then click on the title of this book. Items listed as Student Resources are not password-protected. They include actual patient records in Adobe Portable Document Format (PDF) that students can use to practice coding. (These records are also located in Appendices A-D of the workook.)

Items listed as Instructor Resources are password-protected. To access the protected instructor's content in the online companion (OLC), use the following information:

    Username: greenolc
    Password: enter

> ### Teaching Tip:
>
> *The online companion (OLC) also contains revision files, which include changes to be made in the textbook and/or Instructor's Manual after publication (e.g., revised code numbers due to coding updates). You are welcome to e-mail the authors at delmarauthor@yahoo.com with questions or comments. The authors will respond to your e-mails, and appropriate errata will be posted to the OLC to provide clarification about textbook and workbook content.*

INSTRUCTOR RESOURCE CD-ROM

The Instructor Resource CD-ROM contains an electronic version of this Instructor's Manual, a computerized test bank (CTB), and presentations prepared using Microsoft PowerPoint®. Go to **http://www.delmarhealthcare.com** or contact your Cengage Delmar Learning sales representative to order the Instructor Resource CD-ROM. These same supplements are also on the password-protected side of the Online Companion.

Teaching Tip:

- The CTB contains true/false, short answer, completion, multiple choice, and matching questions. ExamView® software is also included on the Instructor Resource CD-ROM as well as the Online Companion to allow you to generate exams quickly, which can be printed or Web-enabled. This means that you can create different versions of the same exam for large classes of students (when students cannot be separated from each other by an empty desk).

- For online courses, presentations prepared using Microsoft PowerPoint® can be Web-enabled. Just use Microsoft's PowerPoint® software to open a presentation; click "File," then "Save as Web Page." Upload the *.mht file you created to your online course or to the Web. Students do not need Microsoft PowerPoint® software installed on their computer to view the presentation. (If your students have Microsoft PowerPoint® software installed on their computers, you can just upload the *.ppt files to your online course or the Web.)

- An Insurance, Billing, and Coding Curriculum Guide is also located at the Online Companion to assist you in developing new academic programs and in modifying existing programs. The guide contains information about the job outlook and salaries for coders, available professional certification examinations, and curriculum coordination (e.g., marketing, student advising, teaching, professional practices, program approval, and program assessment). Content taught in a coding curriculum is linked to AAPC, AHIMA, and AMBA educational standards. Content is also linked to Cengage Delmar Learning products to assist you in selecting textbooks for instruction. Course outlines and course syllabi are included as samples, and they can be modified for your program. (In Adobe Reader, click on "File," then "Save as Text" to convert the guide to a document that can be opened in word processing software. All of the formatting will be lost, but you can scroll through the document to locate the content you want to cut/paste and modify to reformat. You might find it easier to print pages from the guide, edit them, and then keyboard new documents for your use.)

WEBTUTOR™

WebTutor™ is available as a downloadable course cartridge or e-Pack for schools that use Blackboard, eCollege, WebCT, or another platform (e.g., Angel, Desire2Learn, Educator) as an online learning management system. Go to **http://www.delmarlearning.com/webtutor** to order WebTutor™.

Teaching Tip:

- WebTutor™ can be used to teach a course entirely online or to Web-enhance an on-campus course. (Your textbook author teaches entirely online; but if she ever has an opportunity to teach a face-to-face course again, she will use WebTutor™ to administer all quizzes and exams outside of class time in her college's testing center because that will add five hours or more of teaching time to her courses.)

- Chapter exams in this Instructor's Manual contain the same questions as those included in WebTutor™. Detailed feedback is provided for incorrect answers when students take exams using WebTutor™. (Administering quizzes and exams outside of class time is possible because students are provided with detailed feedback once they submit their quiz or exam. The instructor can delay viewing of detailed feedback until all students have submitted the quiz or exam. For a face-to-face course, the instructor can devote part of a class to discussing the exam results and questions about difficult exam items. For an online course, students can e-mail the instructor or post discussion comments about exam issues.)

SECTION I

Preparing Your Course

3-2-1 Code It! is a comprehensive textbook that covers all coding systems, and its content is written to prepare medical assistants and other health care professionals for beginner or entry-level coding positions. The textbook is organized so that content can be taught in parts (Table 1) in one course as well as in two (or more) courses. Your academic program and course requirements will determine the sections that should be taught to students.

EXAMPLE 1

A sequence of two-semester coding courses could include Parts I and II in an ICD-9-CM coding course. Then Parts III and IV could be taught in a HCPCS/CPT coding course. Many medical assistant and coding programs also teach a separate insurance and reimbursement course, eliminating the need to require Part V in either coding course. However, if your program does not have a separate course, consider adding Part V to one of your coding courses (or to an entirely different course, such as Introduction to Health Information Management).

EXAMPLE 2

A one-semester coding course taught in a medical assistant (MA) or medical office administration (MOA) program could include Parts II, III, and IV, eliminating Chapter 5 from Part II. You could also consider eliminating Chapters 10, 17, and 18 from the course syllabus (and assigning them outside of class or offer them as an independent study course).

Many MA and MOA programs teach a separate insurance and reimbursement course, eliminating the need to include Part V in the coding course. If the program doesn't offer a separate insurance and reimbursement course, consider adding Part V content to a different course (e.g., Administrative Medical Assisting or Introduction to Health Information Management).

Table 1 Organization of *3-2-1 Code It!*

Part	Title	Chapters
I	Coding Overview	Chapter 1: Overview of Coding
II	International Classification of Diseases, Ninth Revision, Clinical Modification (ICD-9-CM) Coding System	Chapter 2: Introduction to ICD-9-CM Coding Chapter 3: ICD-9-CM Coding Conventions Chapter 4: ICD-9-CM Coding Guidelines Chapter 5: ICD-9-CM Hospital Inpatient Coding Chapter 6: ICD-9-CM Outpatient and Physician Office Coding
III	Health Care Procedure Coding System (HCPCS), Level II National Coding System	Chapter 7: HCPCS Level II National Coding System
IV	Current Procedural Terminology (CPT) Coding System	Chapter 8: Introduction to CPT Coding Chapter 9: CPT Evaluation and Management Chapter 10: CPT Anesthesia Chapter 11: CPT Surgery I Chapter 12: CPT Surgery II Chapter 13: CPT Surgery III Chapter 14: CPT Surgery IV Chapter 15: CPT Surgery V Chapter 16: CPT Radiology Chapter 17: CPT Pathology and Laboratory Chapter 18: CPT Medicine
V	Insurance and Reimbursement Overview	Chapter 19: Insurance and Reimbursement

SEMESTER PLANS

The one-semester plan (Table 2) assumes 45 hours of classroom lecture (or 3 hours per week for 15 weeks). Your course may also include an additional 45 hours of laboratory during the semester, for which corresponding workbook chapters can be assigned. The final examination is not included in the 45-hour plan.

Some educators prefer to use this textbook for a two-semester sequential course, teaching ICD-9-CM in one course and HCPCS/CPT in another course. If that is the method you prefer, refer to the two-semester plan (Table 3).

Table 2 One-Semester Plan

Week	Chapter
1–2	Chapter 1: Overview of Coding Chapter 2: Introduction to ICD-9-CM Coding Exam 1
3–4	Chapter 3: ICD-9-CM Coding Conventions Chapter 4: ICD-9-CM Coding Guidelines Exam 2
5–6	Chapter 5: ICD-9-CM Hospital Inpatient Coding Chapter 6: ICD-9-CM Outpatient and Physician Office Coding Exam 3
NOTE: If teaching in a medical assistant or medical office administration program, consider eliminating Chapter 5: ICD-9-CM Inpatient Coding.	
7	Chapter 7: HCPCS Level II National Coding System Exam 4
8	Chapter 8: Introduction to CPT Coding Chapter 10: CPT Anesthesia Exam 5
NOTE: If teaching in a medical assistant or medical office administration program, consider requiring Chapter 10: CPT Anesthesia as an outside-of-class assignment.	
9	Chapter 9: CPT Evaluation and Management Exam 6
10–12	Chapters 11–15: CPT Surgery I–V Exam 7
NOTE: If teaching in a medical assistant or medical office administration program, consider covering just those portions of Chapters 11–15: CPT Surgery I–V that pertain to your academic program's *community of interest*. A *community of interest* includes employers who hire an academic program's graduates; the employers should be surveyed to determine the level of CPT Surgery coding required of graduates. For example, medical assistants might be required to assign codes for simple and intermediate repairs in the CPT Integumentary subsection (but not for skin grafts and flaps, which are often performed in a hospital ambulatory surgery or inpatient setting and coded by hospital outpatient and inpatient coding specialists).	
13–14	Chapter 16: CPT Radiology Chapter 17: CPT Pathology and Laboratory Chapter 18: CPT Medicine Chapter 19: Insurance and Reimbursement Exam 8
15	Review of Chapters 1–19 for final examination
Finals Week	Comprehensive Final Examination (Chapters 1–19)

Table 3 Two-Semester Plan

First Semester

Week	Chapter
1–2	Chapter 1: Overview of Coding Exam 1
3–4	Chapter 2: Introduction to ICD-9-CM Coding Exam 2
5–6	Chapter 3: ICD-9-CM Coding Conventions Exam 3
7–8	Chapter 4: ICD-9-CM Coding Guidelines Exam 4
9–12	Chapter 5: ICD-9-CM Hospital Inpatient Coding Exam 5

NOTE: If teaching in a medical assistant or medical office administration program, consider eliminating Chapter 5: ICD-9-CM Hospital Inpatient Coding (and from Week 15, Review of Chapters 1–6 for final examination and Comprehensive Final Examination).

Week	Chapter
13–14	Chapter 6: ICD-9-CM Outpatient and Physician Office Coding Exam 6
15	Review of Chapters 1–6 for final examination
Finals Week	Comprehensive Final Examination (Chapters 1–6)

Second Semester

Week	Chapter
1	Chapter 7: HCPCS Level II National Coding System Exam 1
2	Chapter 8: Introduction to CPT Coding Exam 2
3–4	Chapter 9: CPT Evaluation and Management Exam 3
5	Chapter 10: CPT Anesthesia Exam 4
6–10	Chapters 11–15: CPT Surgery I–V Exam 5
11	Chapter 16: CPT Radiology Exam 6
12	Chapter 17: CPT Pathology and Laboratory Exam 7
13	Chapter 18: CPT Medicine Exam 8
14	Chapter 19: Insurance and Reimbursement Exam 9

NOTE: If a separate insurance and reimbursement course is taught in your program, consider eliminating Chapter 19: Insurance and Reimbursement (and from Week 15, Review of Chapters 7–19 for final examination and Comprehensive Final Examination).

Week	Chapter
15	Review of Chapters 7–19 for final examination
Finals Week	Comprehensive Final Examination (Chapters 7–19)

ADMINISTERING EXAMS

Administer short quizzes that cover definitions, coding conventions, and so on, to ensure that students keep up with reading assignments. Unit exams include theory and coding practice. If time permits, you may want to include content from the chapter(s) covered in the last unit on the final examination (instead of administering a separate unit exam).

Teaching Tip:

Consider using WebTutor™ to administer quizzes and exams, whether your course is offered entirely online or face-to-face. The detailed feedback for incorrect answers in WebTutor™ will prove helpful to students. If you teach face-to-face, you can administer the online exams in a classroom setting or use your college's testing center. Then devote part of a class to answering students' questions about the exam so they have a good understanding about the concepts they hadn't mastered.

The textbook author enjoys this discussion with students, and she encourages students to challenge the authenticity of questions and answers as a critical thinking activity. When students convince her that a question was badly written or there could have been more than one answer, she rewards them by adding appropriate points to their exam grade. Then, of course, she revises that exam item for future use! This turns what can be an intimidating process, especially for a new instructor, into a fun learning activity for all. Students learn to think critically, new instructors don't dread discussing exam results, and everyone benefits because exam items are revised and perfected each time the course is taught. (As an aside, it can take up to five years for a new instructor to feel totally comfortable discussing exam results. Embracing students' questions and criticisms is a way to jump-start the "road to comfort.")

GRADING ASSIGNMENTS AND EXAMS

It is important to communicate your grading policy for coding assignments and exams. Refer to the suggested grading policies for ICD-9-CM and HCPCS/CPT coding assignments and exams below.

ICD-9-CM Coding

Assign one point for each correct code, including required fourth and fifth digits for diagnosis codes (and required third and fourth digits for procedure codes). Deduct one-half point for each additional code listed that is not required by ICD-9-CM coding principles (e.g., student assigns a code to an inpatient qualified diagnosis and assigns individual codes to its signs and symptoms).

HCPCS and CPT Coding

Assign one point for each correct code, plus one point for each required modifier. Deduct one-half point for each additional code or modifier that is not required by CPT/HCPCS guidelines and notes.

LESSON PLANS

Lesson plans assist instructors in preparing for class so that specific activities and objectives are accomplished. Lesson plans for each textbook chapter have been created to assist you in organizing your course. Just complete the information in the Time row for each chapter; then enter the class and lab numbers to set up your course. (The lesson plans can be used for a one- or two-semester coding course.)

Chapter 1: Overview of Coding

	Task	Resource
Time:	• Instructor preparation (_____ hours) • Introduction to course (1/2 hour) • In-class lecture (_____ hours) • In-class lab (if laboratory component is included as part of course) (_____ hours)	
Topics:	• Career as a Coder • Professional Associations and Discussion Boards • Coding Overview • Documentation as Basis for Coding • Health Data Collection	
Overview:	This chapter focuses on coding career opportunities in health care, the importance of joining professional associations and obtaining coding credentials, the impact of networking with other coding professionals, and the development of opportunities for career advancement. A coding overview provides students with an introduction to coding concepts, including the role patient record documentation plays in accurate coding.	
Objectives:	• Define key terms. • Explain coding career opportunities and the coding credentialing process. • Identify professional associations and describe the benefits of membership. • Clarify student responsibilities during a coding internship. • Identify coding systems used for reimbursement, and indicate the relationship between patient record documentation and accurate coding.	
Prior to class:	• Read textbook and prepare lecture notes. • Review answers to chapter review. • Select workbook assignments for homework. • Prepare course syllabus. • Prepare chapter quiz.	• *3-2-1 Code It!*, Chapter 1 • *Instructor's Manual to Accompany 3-2-1 Code It!*, Chapter 1 • *Workbook to Accompany 3-2-1 Code It!*, Chapter 1 • *Instructor's Manual to Accompany 3-2-1 Code It!*, Introduction • *Instructor's Manual to Accompany 3-2-1 Code It!*, Chapter 1
Class # _____:	• Distribute and explain course syllabus. • Point out major features of textbook. • Review WebTutor™ features (if applicable). • Assign Chapter 1 as reading assignment. • Lecture on Chapter 1 content. • Encourage students to create flash cards. • Assign chapter review as homework.	• Prepared course syllabus • *3-2-1 Code It!*, Preface • *3-2-1 Code It!*, Preface • *3-2-1 Code It!*, Chapter 1 • Lecture notes prepared from *3-2-1 Code!*, Chapter 1 • *3-2-1 Code It!*, Chapter 1 • *3-2-1 Code It!*, Chapter 1
Class # _____:	• Review previous class lecture and answer students' questions about chapter content. • Continue lecture on Chapter 1 content. • Collect homework (and grade). • Administer chapter quiz. • Assign Chapter 1 as reading assignment.	• Ask students to identify key topics and issues from previous class lecture. • *3-2-1 Code It!*, Chapter 1 • *Instructor's Manual to Accompany 3-2-1 Code It!*, Chapter 1 • *Instructor's Manual to Accompany 3-2-1 Code It!*, Chapter 1 • *3-2-1 Code It!*, Chapter 2
Lab # _____:	• Point out major features of workbook. • Communicate assignments to be accomplished during lab and explain how each is to be completed. • Rotate among students as they complete lab assignments to provide individual assistance. • Consider reviewing rough draft work during lab and allowing students to submit final draft at the beginning of the next lab class. • Assign additional workbook assignments for homework.	• *Workbook to Accompany 3-2-1 Code It!*, Preface • *Workbook to Accompany 3-2-1 Code It!*, Chapter 1
Assessment:	• Homework assignments • Chapter quiz • In-class participation • Lab assignments	

Chapter 2: Introduction to ICD-9-CM Coding

Time:	• Instructor preparation (_____ hours) • In-class lecture (_____ hours) • In-class lab (if laboratory component is included as part of course) (_____ hours)
Topics:	• Overview of ICD-9-CM • ICD-9-CM Tabular List of Diseases • ICD-9-CM Index to Diseases • ICD-9-CM Tabular List of Procedures and Index to Procedures • ICD-9-CM Official Guidelines for Coding and Reporting
Overview:	This chapter focuses on the organization of the ICD-9-CM coding system and the official guidelines for coding and reporting.
Objectives:	• Define key terms. • Explain the organization of the ICD-9-CM Tabular List of Diseases, Index to Diseases, and Tabular List of Procedures and Index to Procedures. • List and describe the guidelines for coding and reporting using ICD-9-CM. • Interpret ICD-9-CM guidelines for coding and reporting. • Apply guidelines for coding and reporting when assigning ICD-9-CM codes.

	Task	Resource
Prior to class:	• Read textbook and prepare lecture notes. • Review answers to chapter review. • Select workbook assignments for homework. • Prepare course syllabus. • Prepare chapter quiz.	• *3-2-1 Code It!*, Chapter 2 • *Instructor's Manual to Accompany 3-2-1 Code It!*, Chapter 2 • *Workbook to Accompany 3-2-1 Code It!*, Chapter 2 • *Instructor's Manual to Accompany 3-2-1 Code It!*, Introduction • *Instructor's Manual to Accompany 3-2-1 Code It!*, Chapter 2
Class # ___:	• Distribute and explain course syllabus. • Point out major features of textbook. • Review WebTutor™ features (if applicable). • Assign Chapter 2 as reading assignment. • Lecture on Chapter 2 content. • Encourage students to create flash cards. • Assign chapter review as homework.	• Prepared course syllabus • *3-2-1 Code It!*, Preface • *3-2-1 Code It!*, Preface • *3-2-1 Code It!*, Chapter 2 • Lecture notes prepared from *3-2-1 Code!*, Chapter 2 • *3-2-1 Code It!*, Chapter 2 • *3-2-1 Code It!*, Chapter 2
Class # ___:	• Review previous class lecture and answer students' questions about chapter content. • Continue lecture on Chapter 2 content. • Collect homework (and grade). • Administer chapter quiz. • Assign Chapter 2 as reading assignment.	• Ask students to identify key topics and issues from previous class lecture. • *3-2-1 Code It!*, Chapter 2 • *Instructor's Manual to Accompany 3-2-1 Code It!*, Chapter 2 • *Instructor's Manual to Accompany 3-2-1 Code It!*, Chapter 2 • *3-2-1 Code It!*, Chapter 2
Lab # ___:	• Point out major features of workbook. • Communicate assignments to be accomplished during lab and explain how each is to be completed. • Rotate among students as they complete lab assignments to provide individual assistance. • Consider reviewing rough draft work during lab and allowing students to submit final draft at the beginning of the next lab class. • Assign additional workbook assignments for homework.	• *Workbook to Accompany 3-2-1 Code It!*, Preface • *Workbook to Accompany 3-2-1 Code It!*, Chapter 2
Assessment:	• Homework assignments • Chapter quiz • In-class participation • Lab assignments	

Chapter 3: ICD-9-CM Coding Conventions

Time:	• Instructor preparation (_____ hours) • In-class lecture (_____ hours) • In-class lab (if laboratory component is included as part of course) (_____ hours)
Topics:	• Format • Eponyms • Abbreviations • Punctuation • Boxed Notes • Tables • Includes and Excludes Notes and Inclusion Terms • Other, Other Specified, and Unspecified Codes • Etiology and Manifestation Rules • And • Due to • In • With • Cross-References
Overview:	This chapter focuses on ICD-9-CM coding conventions, which are the rules used when assigning codes.
Objectives:	• Define key terms. • List ICD-9-CM coding conventions. • Explain ICD-9-CM coding conventions. • Identify ICD-9-CM coding conventions as they apply to patient cases. • Interpret ICD-9-CM coding conventions to assign codes accurately.

	Task	Resource
Prior to class:	• Read textbook and prepare lecture notes. • Review answers to chapter review. • Select workbook assignments for homework. • Prepare course syllabus. • Prepare chapter quiz.	• *3-2-1 Code It!*, Chapter 3 • *Instructor's Manual to Accompany 3-2-1 Code It!*, Chapter 3 • *Workbook to Accompany 3-2-1 Code It!*, Chapter 3 • *Instructor's Manual to Accompany 3-2-1 Code It!*, Introduction • *Instructor's Manual to Accompany 3-2-1 Code It!*, Chapter 3
Class # ___:	• Distribute and explain course syllabus. • Point out major features of textbook. • Review WebTutor™ features (if applicable). • Assign Chapter 3 as reading assignment. • Lecture on Chapter 3 content. • Encourage students to create flash cards. • Assign chapter review as homework.	• Prepared course syllabus • *3-2-1 Code It!*, Preface • *3-2-1 Code It!*, Preface • *3-2-1 Code It!*, Chapter 3 • Lecture notes prepared from *3-2-1 Code!*, Chapter 3 • *3-2-1 Code It!*, Chapter 3 • *3-2-1 Code It!*, Chapter 3
Class # ___:	• Review previous class lecture and answer students' questions about chapter content. • Continue lecture on Chapter 3 content. • Collect homework (and grade). • Administer chapter quiz. • Assign Chapter 3 as reading assignment.	• Ask students to identify key topics and issues from previous class lecture. • *3-2-1 Code It!*, Chapter 3 • *Instructor's Manual to Accompany 3-2-1 Code It!*, Chapter 3 • *Instructor's Manual to Accompany 3-2-1 Code It!*, Chapter 3 • *3-2-1 Code It!*, Chapter 3
Lab # ___:	• Point out major features of workbook. • Communicate assignments to be accomplished during lab and explain how each is to be completed. • Rotate among students as they complete lab assignments to provide individual assistance. • Consider reviewing rough draft work during lab and allowing students to submit final draft at the beginning of the next lab class. • Assign additional workbook assignments for homework.	• *Workbook to Accompany 3-2-1 Code It!*, Preface • *Workbook to Accompany 3-2-1 Code It!*, Chapter 3
Assessment:	• Homework assignments • Chapter quiz • In-class participation • Lab assignments	

Chapter 4: ICD-9-CM Coding Guidelines

Time:	• Instructor preparation (_____ hours) • In-class lecture (_____ hours) • In-class lab (if laboratory component is included as part of course) (_____ hours)
Topics:	• ICD-9-CM Official Guidelines for Coding and Reporting • General ICD-9-CM Diagnosis Coding Guidelines • General ICD-9-CM Procedure Coding Guidelines • ICD-9-CM Chapter-Specific Coding Guidelines
Overview:	This chapter focuses on the interpretation of the *Guidelines for Coding and Reporting Using ICD-9-CM*, including general ICD-9-CM diagnosis coding guidelines, general ICD-9-CM procedure coding guidelines, and ICD-9-CM chapter-specific coding guidelines.
Objectives:	• Define key terms. • Explain HIPAA's impact on the adherence to *ICD-9-CM Official Guidelines for Coding and Reporting.* • Describe the content of each section of the *ICD-9-CM Official Guidelines for Coding and Reporting.* • Apply general ICD-9-CM coding guidelines when assigning codes to diagnoses and procedures. • Apply chapter-specific ICD-9-CM coding guidelines when assigning codes to diagnoses.

	Task	Resource
Prior to class:	• Read textbook and prepare lecture notes. • Review answers to chapter review. • Select workbook assignments for homework. • Prepare course syllabus. • Prepare chapter quiz.	• *3-2-1 Code It!*, Chapter 4 • *Instructor's Manual to Accompany 3-2-1 Code It!*, Chapter 4 • *Workbook to Accompany 3-2-1 Code It!*, Chapter 4 • *Instructor's Manual to Accompany 3-2-1 Code It!*, Introduction • *Instructor's Manual to Accompany 3-2-1 Code It!*, Chapter 4
Class # ___:	• Distribute and explain course syllabus. • Point out major features of textbook. • Review WebTutor™ features (if applicable). • Assign Chapter 4 as reading assignment. • Lecture on Chapter 4 content. • Encourage students to create flash cards. • Assign chapter review as homework.	• Prepared course syllabus • *3-2-1 Code It!*, Preface • *3-2-1 Code It!*, Preface • *3-2-1 Code It!*, Chapter 4 • Lecture notes prepared from *3-2-1 Code It!*, Chapter 4 • *3-2-1 Code It!*, Chapter 4 • *3-2-1 Code It!*, Chapter 4
Class # ___:	• Review previous class lecture and answer students' questions about chapter content. • Continue lecture on Chapter 4 content. • Collect homework (and grade). • Administer chapter quiz. • Assign Chapter 4 as reading assignment.	• Ask students to identify key topics and issues from previous class lecture. • *3-2-1 Code It!*, Chapter 4 • *Instructor's Manual to Accompany 3-2-1 Code It!*, Chapter 4 • *Instructor's Manual to Accompany 3-2-1 Code It!*, Chapter 4 • *3-2-1 Code It!*, Chapter 4
Lab # ___:	• Point out major features of workbook. • Communicate assignments to be accomplished during lab and explain how each is to be completed. • Rotate among students as they complete lab assignments to provide individual assistance. • Consider reviewing rough draft work during lab and allowing students to submit final draft at the beginning of the next lab class. • Assign additional workbook assignments for homework.	• *Workbook to Accompany 3-2-1 Code It!*, Preface • *Workbook to Accompany 3-2-1 Code It!*, Chapter 4
Assessment:	• Homework assignments • Chapter quiz • In-class participation • Lab assignments	

Chapter 5: ICD-9-CM Hospital Inpatient Coding

Time:	• Instructor preparation (_____ hours) • In-class lecture (_____ hours) • In-class lab (if laboratory component is included as part of course) (_____ hours)
Topics:	• Acute Care Facilities (Hospitals) • Inpatient Coding Guidelines
Overview:	This chapter focuses on inpatient acute care settings (e.g., hospitals) and includes an interpretation of guidelines for sequencing diagnoses and procedures, which are published in the *Guidelines for Coding and Reporting Using ICD-9-CM* and used as a companion to the official version of ICD-9-CM.
Objectives:	• Define key terms. • List and explain differences among acute care inpatient settings. • Interpret inpatient diagnosis and procedure coding and reporting guidelines. • Assign ICD-9-CM diagnosis and/or procedure codes for acute care inpatient cases.

	Task	Resource
Prior to class:	• Read textbook and prepare lecture notes. • Review answers to chapter review. • Select workbook assignments for homework. • Prepare course syllabus. • Prepare chapter quiz.	• *3-2-1 Code It!*, Chapter 5 • *Instructor's Manual to Accompany 3-2-1 Code It!*, Chapter 5 • *Workbook to Accompany 3-2-1 Code It!*, Chapter 5 • *Instructor's Manual to Accompany 3-2-1 Code It!*, Introduction • *Instructor's Manual to Accompany 3-2-1 Code It!*, Chapter 5
Class # ___:	• Distribute and explain course syllabus. • Point out major features of textbook. • Review WebTutor™ features (if applicable). • Assign Chapter 5 as reading assignment. • Lecture on Chapter 5 content. • Encourage students to create flash cards. • Assign chapter review as homework.	• Prepared course syllabus • *3-2-1 Code It!*, Preface • *3-2-1 Code It!*, Preface • *3-2-1 Code It!*, Chapter 5 • Lecture notes prepared from *3-2-1 Code!*, Chapter 5 • *3-2-1 Code It!*, Chapter 5 • *3-2-1 Code It!*, Chapter 5
Class # ___:	• Review previous class lecture and answer students' questions about chapter content. • Continue lecture on Chapter 5 content. • Collect homework (and grade). • Administer chapter quiz. • Assign Chapter 5 as reading assignment.	• Ask students to identify key topics and issues from previous class lecture. • *3-2-1 Code It!*, Chapter 5 • *Instructor's Manual to Accompany 3-2-1 Code It!*, Chapter 5 • *Instructor's Manual to Accompany 3-2-1 Code It!*, Chapter 5 • *3-2-1 Code It!*, Chapter 5
Lab # ___:	• Point out major features of workbook. • Communicate assignments to be accomplished during lab and explain how each is to be completed. • Rotate among students as they complete lab assignments to provide individual assistance. • Consider reviewing rough draft work during lab and allowing students to submit final draft at the beginning of the next lab class. • Assign additional workbook assignments for homework.	• *Workbook to Accompany 3-2-1 Code It!*, Preface • *Workbook to Accompany 3-2-1 Code It!*, Chapter 5
Assessment:	• Homework assignments • Chapter quiz • In-class participation • Lab assignments	

Chapter 6: ICD-9-CM Outpatient and Physician Office Coding

Time:	• Instructor preparation (_____ hours) • In-class lecture (_____ hours) • In-class lab (if laboratory component is included as part of course) (_____ hours)
Topics:	• Outpatient Care • Diagnostic Coding and Reporting Guidelines for Outpatient Services: Hospital-Based and Physician Office • ICD-9-CM Coding Guidelines for Outpatient Diagnostic Tests
Overview:	This chapter focuses on outpatient care and physician office settings and interprets the *Diagnostic Coding and Reporting Guidelines for Outpatient Services: Hospital-Based and Physician Office.*
Objectives:	• Define key terms. • List and explain differences among outpatient and physician office health care settings. • Interpret outpatient diagnosis coding and reporting guidelines. • Assign ICD-9-CM diagnosis codes for outpatient and physician office care.

	Task	Resource
Prior to class:	• Read textbook and prepare lecture notes. • Review answers to chapter review. • Select workbook assignments for homework. • Prepare course syllabus. • Prepare chapter quiz.	• *3-2-1 Code It!*, Chapter 6 • *Instructor's Manual to Accompany 3-2-1 Code It!*, Chapter 6 • *Workbook to Accompany 3-2-1 Code It!*, Chapter 6 • *Instructor's Manual to Accompany 3-2-1 Code It!*, Introduction • *Instructor's Manual to Accompany 3-2-1 Code It!*, Chapter 6
Class # ___:	• Distribute and explain course syllabus. • Point out major features of textbook. • Review WebTutor™ features (if applicable). • Assign Chapter 6 as reading assignment. • Lecture on Chapter 6 content. • Encourage students to create flash cards. • Assign chapter review as homework.	• Prepared course syllabus • *3-2-1 Code It!*, Preface • *3-2-1 Code It!*, Preface • *3-2-1 Code It!*, Chapter 6 • Lecture notes prepared from *3-2-1 Code!*, Chapter 6 • *3-2-1 Code It!*, Chapter 6 • *3-2-1 Code It!*, Chapter 6
Class # ___:	• Review previous class lecture and answer students' questions about chapter content. • Continue lecture on Chapter 6 content. • Collect homework (and grade). • Administer chapter quiz. • Assign Chapter 6 as reading assignment.	• Ask students to identify key topics and issues from previous class lecture. • *3-2-1 Code It!*, Chapter 6 • *Instructor's Manual to Accompany 3-2-1 Code It!*, Chapter 6 • *Instructor's Manual to Accompany 3-2-1 Code It!*, Chapter 6 • *3-2-1 Code It!*, Chapter 6
Lab # ___:	• Point out major features of workbook. • Communicate assignments to be accomplished during lab and explain how each is to be completed. • Rotate among students as they complete lab assignments to provide individual assistance. • Consider reviewing rough draft work during lab and allowing students to submit final draft at the beginning of the next lab class. • Assign additional workbook assignments for homework.	• *Workbook to Accompany 3-2-1 Code It!*, Preface • *Workbook to Accompany 3-2-1 Code It!*, Chapter 6
Assessment:	• Homework assignments • Chapter quiz • In-class participation • Lab assignments	

Chapter 7: HCPCS Level II National Coding System

Time:	• Instructor preparation (_____ hours) • In-class lecture (_____ hours) • In-class lab (if laboratory component is included as part of course) (_____ hours)
Topics:	• Overview of HCPCS • Assigning HCPCS Level II Codes • Determining Payer Responsibility
Overview:	This chapter focuses on the HCPCS level II national coding system, which contains alphanumeric codes that were developed to complement the *Current Procedural Terminology* (CPT) coding system.
Objectives:	• Define key terms. • List the HCPCS levels and their components. • Assign HCPCS level II procedure and services codes for outpatient care. • Identify situations in which both HCPCS levels I and II codes are assigned. • Assign claims to primary Medicare administrative contractor (MACs) or Durable Medical Equipment MACs according to HCPCS level II code number.

	Task	Resource
Prior to class:	• Read textbook and prepare lecture notes. • Review answers to chapter review. • Select workbook assignments for homework. • Prepare course syllabus. • Prepare chapter quiz.	• *3-2-1 Code It!*, Chapter 7 • *Instructor's Manual to Accompany 3-2-1 Code It!*, Chapter 7 • *Workbook to Accompany 3-2-1 Code It!*, Chapter 7 • *Instructor's Manual to Accompany 3-2-1 Code It!*, Introduction • *Instructor's Manual to Accompany 3-2-1 Code It!*, Chapter 7
Class # ____:	• Distribute and explain course syllabus. • Point out major features of textbook. • Review WebTutor™ features (if applicable). • Assign Chapter 7 as reading assignment. • Lecture on Chapter 7 content. • Encourage students to create flash cards. • Assign chapter review as homework.	• Prepared course syllabus • *3-2-1 Code It!*, Preface • *3-2-1 Code It!*, Preface • *3-2-1 Code It!*, Chapter 7 • Lecture notes prepared from *3-2-1 Code!*, Chapter 7 • *3-2-1 Code It!*, Chapter 7 • *3-2-1 Code It!*, Chapter 7
Class # ____:	• Review previous class lecture and answer students' questions about chapter content. • Continue lecture on Chapter 7 content. • Collect homework (and grade). • Administer chapter quiz. • Assign Chapter 7 as reading assignment.	• Ask students to identify key topics and issues from previous class lecture. • *3-2-1 Code It!*, Chapter 7 • *Instructor's Manual to Accompany 3-2-1 Code It!*, Chapter 7 • *Instructor's Manual to Accompany 3-2-1 Code It!*, Chapter 7 • *3-2-1 Code It!*, Chapter 7
Lab # ____:	• Point out major features of workbook. • Communicate assignments to be accomplished during lab and explain how each is to be completed. • Rotate among students as they complete lab assignments to provide individual assistance. • Consider reviewing rough draft work during lab and allowing students to submit final draft at the beginning of the next lab class. • Assign additional workbook assignments for homework.	• *Workbook to Accompany 3-2-1 Code It!*, Preface • *Workbook to Accompany 3-2-1 Code It!*, Chapter 7
Assessment:	• Homework assignments • Chapter quiz • In-class participation • Lab assignments	

Chapter 8: Introduction to CPT Coding

Time:	• Instructor preparation (_____ hours) • In-class lecture (_____ hours) • In-class lab (if laboratory component is included as part of course) (_____ hours)
Topics:	• History of CPT • Overview of CPT • Organization of CPT • CPT Index • CPT Appendices • CPT Symbols • CPT Sections, Subsections, Categories, and Subcategories • CPT Modifiers • National Correct Coding Initiative (NCCI)
Overview:	This chapter introduces the *Current Procedural Terminology* (CPT) coding system (or HCPCS level I).
Objectives:	• Define key terms. • Explain the organization, format, and content of CPT. • Interpret CPT section guidelines, coding notes, and modifiers. • Assign CPT procedure and service codes for outpatient care. • Add CPT and/or HCPCS level II modifiers to codes as appropriate.

	Task	Resource
Prior to class:	• Read textbook and prepare lecture notes. • Review answers to chapter review. • Select workbook assignments for homework. • Prepare course syllabus. • Prepare chapter quiz.	• *3-2-1 Code It!*, Chapter 8 • *Instructor's Manual to Accompany 3-2-1 Code It!*, Chapter 8 • *Workbook to Accompany 3-2-1 Code It!*, Chapter 8 • *Instructor's Manual to Accompany 3-2-1 Code It!*, Introduction • *Instructor's Manual to Accompany 3-2-1 Code It!*, Chapter 8
Class # ____:	• Distribute and explain course syllabus. • Point out major features of textbook. • Review WebTutor™ features (if applicable). • Assign Chapter 8 as reading assignment. • Lecture on Chapter 8 content. • Encourage students to create flash cards. • Assign chapter review as homework.	• Prepared course syllabus • *3-2-1 Code It!*, Preface • *3-2-1 Code It!*, Preface • *3-2-1 Code It!*, Chapter 8 • Lecture notes prepared from *3-2-1 Code!*, Chapter 8 • *3-2-1 Code It!*, Chapter 8 • *3-2-1 Code It!*, Chapter 8
Class # ____:	• Review previous class lecture and answer students' questions about chapter content. • Continue lecture on Chapter 8 content. • Collect homework (and grade). • Administer chapter quiz. • Assign Chapter 8 as reading assignment.	• Ask students to identify key topics and issues from previous class lecture. • *3-2-1 Code It!*, Chapter 8 • *Instructor's Manual to Accompany 3-2-1 Code It!*, Chapter 8 • *Instructor's Manual to Accompany 3-2-1 Code It!*, Chapter 8 • *3-2-1 Code It!*, Chapter 8
Lab # ___:	• Point out major features of workbook. • Communicate assignments to be accomplished during lab and explain how each is to be completed. • Rotate among students as they complete lab assignments to provide individual assistance. • Consider reviewing rough draft work during lab and allowing students to submit final draft at the beginning of the next lab class. • Assign additional workbook assignments for homework.	• *Workbook to Accompany 3-2-1 Code It!*, Preface • *Workbook to Accompany 3-2-1 Code It!*, Chapter 8
Assessment:	• Homework assignments • Chapter quiz • In-class participation • Lab assignments	

Chapter 9: CPT Evaluation and Management

Time:	• Instructor preparation (_____ hours) • In-class lecture (_____ hours) • In-class lab (if laboratory component is included as part of course) (_____ hours)
Topics:	• Overview of Evaluation and Management Section • Evaluation and Management Section Guidelines • Levels of Evaluation and Management Services • Evaluation and Management Categories and Subcategories
Overview:	This chapter focuses on CPT evaluation and management codes, which generate most of the revenue for the physician's office.
Objectives:	• Define key terms. • Explain the organization, format, and content of the CPT Evaluation and Management section. • Interpret CPT Evaluation and Management section guidelines, coding notes, and modifiers. • Select CPT evaluation and management levels of service for documented patient care. • Assign CPT evaluation and management service codes for patient care. • Add CPT and/or HCPCS level II modifiers to codes as appropriate.

	Task	Resource
Prior to class:	• Read textbook and prepare lecture notes. • Review answers to chapter review. • Select workbook assignments for homework. • Prepare course syllabus. • Prepare chapter quiz.	• *3-2-1 Code It!*, Chapter 9 • *Instructor's Manual to Accompany 3-2-1 Code It!*, Chapter 9 • *Workbook to Accompany 3-2-1 Code It!*, Chapter 9 • *Instructor's Manual to Accompany 3-2-1 Code It!*, Introduction • *Instructor's Manual to Accompany 3-2-1 Code It!*, Chapter 9
Class # ___:	• Distribute and explain course syllabus. • Point out major features of textbook. • Review WebTutor™ features (if applicable). • Assign Chapter 9 as reading assignment. • Lecture on Chapter 9 content. • Encourage students to create flash cards. • Assign chapter review as homework.	• Prepared course syllabus • *3-2-1 Code It!*, Preface • *3-2-1 Code It!*, Preface • *3-2-1 Code It!*, Chapter 9 • Lecture notes prepared from *3-2-1 Code!*, Chapter 9 • *3-2-1 Code It!*, Chapter 9 • *3-2-1 Code It!*, Chapter 9
Class # ___:	• Review previous class lecture and answer students' questions about chapter content. • Continue lecture on Chapter 9 content. • Collect homework (and grade). • Administer chapter quiz. • Assign Chapter 9 as reading assignment.	• Ask students to identify key topics and issues from previous class lecture. • *3-2-1 Code It!*, Chapter 9 • *Instructor's Manual to Accompany 3-2-1 Code It!*, Chapter 9 • *Instructor's Manual to Accompany 3-2-1 Code It!*, Chapter 9 • *3-2-1 Code It!*, Chapter 9
Lab # ___:	• Point out major features of workbook. • Communicate assignments to be accomplished during lab and explain how each is to be completed. • Rotate among students as they complete lab assignments to provide individual assistance. • Consider reviewing rough draft work during lab and allowing students to submit final draft at the beginning of the next lab class. • Assign additional workbook assignments for homework.	• *Workbook to Accompany 3-2-1 Code It!*, Preface • *Workbook to Accompany 3-2-1 Code It!*, Chapter 9
Assessment:	• Homework assignments • Chapter quiz • In-class participation • Lab assignments	

Chapter 10: CPT Anesthesia

Time:	• Instructor preparation (_____ hours) • In-class lecture (_____ hours) • In-class lab (if laboratory component is included as part of course) (_____ hours)
Topics:	• Anesthesia Terminology • Overview of Anesthesia Section • Anesthesia Section Guidelines • Anesthesia Subsections
Overview:	This chapter focuses on CPT anesthesia codes, which are reported for services related to the administration of anesthesia (including general and regional), the supplementation of local anesthesia, and other supportive anesthesia services.
Objectives:	• Define key terms. • Explain the organization, format, and content of the CPT Anesthesia section. • Interpret CPT anesthesia section guidelines, coding notes, and modifiers. • Assign CPT evaluation and management service codes. • Add CPT and/or HCPCS level II modifiers to codes as appropriate. • Calculate anesthesia fees.

	Task	Resource
Prior to class:	• Read textbook and prepare lecture notes. • Review answers to chapter review. • Select workbook assignments for homework. • Prepare course syllabus. • Prepare chapter quiz.	• *3-2-1 Code It!*, Chapter 10 • *Instructor's Manual to Accompany 3-2-1 Code It!*, Chapter 10 • *Workbook to Accompany 3-2-1 Code It!*, Chapter 10 • *Instructor's Manual to Accompany 3-2-1 Code It!*, Introduction • *Instructor's Manual to Accompany 3-2-1 Code It!*, Chapter 10
Class # ___:	• Distribute and explain course syllabus. • Point out major features of textbook. • Review WebTutor™ features (if applicable). • Assign Chapter 10 as reading assignment. • Lecture on Chapter 10 content. • Encourage students to create flash cards. • Assign chapter review as homework.	• Prepared course syllabus • *3-2-1 Code It!*, Preface • *3-2-1 Code It!*, Preface • *3-2-1 Code It!*, Chapter 10 • Lecture notes prepared from *3-2-1 Code!*, Chapter 10 • *3-2-1 Code It!*, Chapter 10 • *3-2-1 Code It!*, Chapter 10
Class # ___:	• Review previous class lecture and answer students' questions about chapter content. • Continue lecture on Chapter 10 content. • Collect homework (and grade). • Administer chapter quiz. • Assign Chapter 10 as reading assignment.	• Ask students to identify key topics and issues from previous class lecture. • *3-2-1 Code It!*, Chapter 10 • *Instructor's Manual to Accompany 3-2-1 Code It!*, Chapter 10 • *Instructor's Manual to Accompany 3-2-1 Code It!*, Chapter 10 • *3-2-1 Code It!*, Chapter 10
Lab # ___:	• Point out major features of workbook. • Communicate assignments to be accomplished during lab and explain how each is to be completed. • Rotate among students as they complete lab assignments to provide individual assistance. • Consider reviewing rough draft work during lab and allowing students to submit final draft at the beginning of the next lab class. • Assign additional workbook assignments for homework.	• *Workbook to Accompany 3-2-1 Code It!*, Preface • *Workbook to Accompany 3-2-1 Code It!*, Chapter 10
Assessment:	• Homework assignments • Chapter quiz • In-class participation • Lab assignments	

Chapter 11: CPT Surgery I

Time:	• Instructor preparation (_____ hours) • In-class lecture (_____ hours) • In-class lab (if laboratory component is included as part of course) (_____ hours)
Topics:	• Overview of Surgery Section • Surgery Guidelines • General Subsection • Integumentary System Subsection
Overview:	This chapter provides an overview of the CPT Surgery section and covers its guidelines. The chapter also focuses on the CPT Surgery General and Integumentary System subsections.
Objectives:	• Define key terms. • Explain the organization, format, and content of the CPT Surgery section. • Interpret CPT Surgery section guidelines and modifiers • Interpret CPT surgery coding notes for the General and Integumentary System subsections. • Assign CPT surgery codes from the General and Integumentary System subsections. • Add CPT and/or HCPCS level II modifiers to codes as appropriate.

	Task	Resource
Prior to class:	• Read textbook and prepare lecture notes. • Review answers to chapter review. • Select workbook assignments for homework. • Prepare course syllabus. • Prepare chapter quiz.	• *3-2-1 Code It!*, Chapter 11 • *Instructor's Manual to Accompany 3-2-1 Code It!*, Chapter 11 • *Workbook to Accompany 3-2-1 Code It!*, Chapter 11 • *Instructor's Manual to Accompany 3-2-1 Code It!*, Introduction • *Instructor's Manual to Accompany 3-2-1 Code It!*, Chapter 11
Class # ___:	• Distribute and explain course syllabus. • Point out major features of textbook. • Review WebTutor™ features (if applicable). • Assign Chapter 11 as reading assignment. • Lecture on Chapter 11 content. • Encourage students to create flash cards. • Assign chapter review as homework.	• Prepared course syllabus • *3-2-1 Code It!*, Preface • *3-2-1 Code It!*, Preface • *3-2-1 Code It!*, Chapter 11 • Lecture notes prepared from *3-2-1 Code!*, Chapter 11 • *3-2-1 Code It!*, Chapter 11 • *3-2-1 Code It!*, Chapter 11
Class # ___:	• Review previous class lecture and answer students' questions about chapter content. • Continue lecture on Chapter 11 content. • Collect homework (and grade). • Administer chapter quiz. • Assign Chapter 11 as reading assignment.	• Ask students to identify key topics and issues from previous class lecture. • *3-2-1 Code It!*, Chapter 11 • *Instructor's Manual to Accompany 3-2-1 Code It!*, Chapter 11 • *Instructor's Manual to Accompany 3-2-1 Code It!*, Chapter 11 • *3-2-1 Code It!*, Chapter 11
Lab # ___:	• Point out major features of workbook. • Communicate assignments to be accomplished during lab and explain how each is to be completed. • Rotate among students as they complete lab assignments to provide individual assistance. • Consider reviewing rough draft work during lab and allowing students to submit final draft at the beginning of the next lab class. • Assign additional workbook assignments for homework.	• *Workbook to Accompany 3-2-1 Code It!*, Preface • *Workbook to Accompany 3-2-1 Code It!*, Chapter 11
Assessment:	• Homework assignments • Chapter quiz • In-class participation • Lab assignments	

Chapter 12: CPT Surgery II

Time:	• Instructor preparation (_____ hours)
	• In-class lecture (_____ hours)
	• In-class lab (if laboratory component is included as part of course) (_____ hours)

Topics:	• Musculoskeletal System Subsection
	• Respiratory System Subsection

Overview:	This chapter focuses on the CPT Surgery Musculoskeletal System and Respiratory System subsections.

Objectives:	• Define key terms.
	• Explain the organization, format, and content of the CPT Surgery Musculoskeletal and Respiratory subsections.
	• Interpret CPT surgery coding notes for the Musculoskeletal and Respiratory System subsections.
	• Assign CPT surgery codes from the Musculoskeletal and Respiratory System Integumentary subsections.
	• Add CPT and/or HCPCS level II modifiers to codes as appropriate.

	Task	Resource
Prior to class:	• Read textbook and prepare lecture notes.	• *3-2-1 Code It!*, Chapter 12
	• Review answers to chapter review.	• *Instructor's Manual to Accompany 3-2-1 Code It!*, Chapter 12
	• Select workbook assignments for homework.	• *Workbook to Accompany 3-2-1 Code It!*, Chapter 12
	• Prepare course syllabus.	
	• Prepare chapter quiz.	• *Instructor's Manual to Accompany 3-2-1 Code It!*, Introduction
		• *Instructor's Manual to Accompany 3-2-1 Code It!*, Chapter 12
Class # ___:	• Distribute and explain course syllabus.	• Prepared course syllabus
	• Point out major features of textbook.	• *3-2-1 Code It!*, Preface
	• Review WebTutor™ features (if applicable).	• *3-2-1 Code It!*, Preface
	• Assign Chapter 12 as reading assignment.	• *3-2-1 Code It!*, Chapter 12
	• Lecture on Chapter 12 content.	• Lecture notes prepared from *3-2-1 Code!*, Chapter 12
	• Encourage students to create flash cards.	• *3-2-1 Code It!*, Chapter 12
	• Assign chapter review as homework.	• *3-2-1 Code It!*, Chapter 12
Class # ___:	• Review previous class lecture and answer students' questions about chapter content.	• Ask students to identify key topics and issues from previous class lecture.
	• Continue lecture on Chapter 12 content.	• *3-2-1 Code It!*, Chapter 12
	• Collect homework (and grade).	• *Instructor's Manual to Accompany 3-2-1 Code It!*, Chapter 12
	• Administer chapter quiz.	
	• Assign Chapter 12 as reading assignment.	• *Instructor's Manual to Accompany 3-2-1 Code It!*, Chapter 12
		• *3-2-1 Code It!*, Chapter 12
Lab # ___:	• Point out major features of workbook.	• *Workbook to Accompany 3-2-1 Code It!*, Preface
	• Communicate assignments to be accomplished during lab and explain how each is to be completed.	• *Workbook to Accompany 3-2-1 Code It!*, Chapter 12
	• Rotate among students as they complete lab assignments to provide individual assistance.	
	• Consider reviewing rough draft work during lab and allowing students to submit final draft at the beginning of the next lab class.	
	• Assign additional workbook assignments for homework.	
Assessment:	• Homework assignments	
	• Chapter quiz	
	• In-class participation	
	• Lab assignments	

Chapter 13: CPT Surgery III

Time:	• Instructor preparation (_____ hours) • In-class lecture (_____ hours) • In-class lab (if laboratory component is included as part of course) (_____ hours)	
Topics:	• Cardiovascular System Subsection • Hemic and Lymphatic Systems Subsection	
Overview:	This chapter focuses on the CPT Surgery Cardiovascular System and Hemic and Lymphatic Systems subsections.	
Objectives:	• Define key terms. • Explain the organization, format, and content of the CPT Surgery Cardiovascular System and Hemic and Lymphatic Systems subsections. • Interpret CPT surgery coding notes for the Cardiovascular System and Hemic and Lymphatic Systems subsections. • Assign CPT surgery codes from the Cardiovascular System and Hemic and Lymphatic Systems subsections. • Add CPT and/or HCPCS level II modifiers to codes as appropriate.	

	Task	Resource
Prior to class:	• Read textbook and prepare lecture notes. • Review answers to chapter review. • Select workbook assignments for homework. • Prepare course syllabus. • Prepare chapter quiz.	• *3-2-1 Code It!*, Chapter 13 • *Instructor's Manual to Accompany 3-2-1 Code It!*, Chapter 13 • *Workbook to Accompany 3-2-1 Code It!*, Chapter 13 • *Instructor's Manual to Accompany 3-2-1 Code It!*, Introduction • *Instructor's Manual to Accompany 3-2-1 Code It!*, Chapter 13
Class # ___:	• Distribute and explain course syllabus. • Point out major features of textbook. • Review WebTutor™ features (if applicable). • Assign Chapter 13 as reading assignment. • Lecture on Chapter 13 content. • Encourage students to create flash cards. • Assign chapter review as homework.	• Prepared course syllabus • *3-2-1 Code It!*, Preface • *3-2-1 Code It!*, Preface • *3-2-1 Code It!*, Chapter 13 • Lecture notes prepared from *3-2-1 Code!*, Chapter 13 • *3-2-1 Code It!*, Chapter 13 • *3-2-1 Code It!*, Chapter 13
Class # ___:	• Review previous class lecture and answer students' questions about chapter content. • Continue lecture on Chapter 13 content. • Collect homework (and grade). • Administer chapter quiz. • Assign Chapter 13 as reading assignment.	• Ask students to identify key topics and issues from previous class lecture. • *3-2-1 Code It!*, Chapter 13 • *Instructor's Manual to Accompany 3-2-1 Code It!*, Chapter 13 • *Instructor's Manual to Accompany 3-2-1 Code It!*, Chapter 13 • *3-2-1 Code It!*, Chapter 13
Lab # ___:	• Point out major features of workbook. • Communicate assignments to be accomplished during lab and explain how each is to be completed. • Rotate among students as they complete lab assignments to provide individual assistance. • Consider reviewing rough draft work during lab and allowing students to submit final draft at the beginning of the next lab class. • Assign additional workbook assignments for homework.	• *Workbook to Accompany 3-2-1 Code It!*, Preface • *Workbook to Accompany 3-2-1 Code It!*, Chapter 13
Assessment:	• Homework assignments • Chapter quiz • In-class participation • Lab assignments	

Chapter 14: CPT Surgery IV

Time:	• Instructor preparation (_____ hours)
	• In-class lecture (_____ hours)
	• In-class lab (if laboratory component is included as part of course) (_____ hours)
Topics:	• Mediastinum and Diaphragm Subsection
	• Digestive System Subsection
	• Urinary System Subsection
Overview:	This chapter focuses on the CPT Surgery Mediastinum and Diaphragm, Digestive System, and Urinary System subsections.
Objectives:	• Define key terms.
	• Explain the organization, format, and content of the CPT Mediastinum and Diaphragm, Digestive System, and Urinary System subsections.
	• Interpret CPT surgery coding notes for the Mediastinum and Diaphragm, Digestive System, and Urinary System subsections.
	• Assign CPT surgery codes from the Mediastinum and Diaphragm, Digestive System, and Urinary System subsections.
	• Add CPT and/or HCPCS level II modifiers to codes as appropriate.

	Task	Resource
Prior to class:	• Read textbook and prepare lecture notes.	• *3-2-1 Code It!*, Chapter 14
	• Review answers to chapter review.	• *Instructor's Manual to Accompany 3-2-1 Code It!*, Chapter 14
	• Select workbook assignments for homework.	• *Workbook to Accompany 3-2-1 Code It!*, Chapter 14
	• Prepare course syllabus.	• *Instructor's Manual to Accompany 3-2-1 Code It!*, Introduction
	• Prepare chapter quiz.	• *Instructor's Manual to Accompany 3-2-1 Code It!*, Chapter 14
Class # ___:	• Distribute and explain course syllabus.	• Prepared course syllabus
	• Point out major features of textbook.	• *3-2-1 Code It!*, Preface
	• Review WebTutor™ features (if applicable).	• *3-2-1 Code It!*, Preface
	• Assign Chapter 14 as reading assignment.	• *3-2-1 Code It!*, Chapter 14
	• Lecture on Chapter 14 content.	• Lecture notes prepared from *3-2-1 Code!*, Chapter 14
	• Encourage students to create flash cards.	• *3-2-1 Code It!*, Chapter 14
	• Assign chapter review as homework.	• *3-2-1 Code It!*, Chapter 14
Class # ___:	• Review previous class lecture and answer students' questions about chapter content.	• Ask students to identify key topics and issues from previous class lecture.
	• Continue lecture on Chapter 14 content.	• *3-2-1 Code It!*, Chapter 14
	• Collect homework (and grade).	• *Instructor's Manual to Accompany 3-2-1 Code It!*, Chapter 14
	• Administer chapter quiz.	• *Instructor's Manual to Accompany 3-2-1 Code It!*, Chapter 14
	• Assign Chapter 14 as reading assignment.	• *3-2-1 Code It!*, Chapter 14
Lab # ___:	• Point out major features of workbook.	• *Workbook to Accompany 3-2-1 Code It!*, Preface
	• Communicate assignments to be accomplished during lab and explain how each is to be completed.	• *Workbook to Accompany 3-2-1 Code It!*, Chapter 14
	• Rotate among students as they complete lab assignments to provide individual assistance.	
	• Consider reviewing rough draft work during lab and allowing students to submit final draft at the beginning of the next lab class.	
	• Assign additional workbook assignments for homework.	
Assessment:	• Homework assignments	
	• Chapter quiz	
	• In-class participation	
	• Lab assignments	

Chapter 15: CPT Surgery V

Time:	• Instructor preparation (_____ hours) • In-class lecture (_____ hours) • In-class lab (if laboratory component is included as part of course) (_____ hours)
Topics:	• Male Genital System Subsection • Reproductive System Procedures Subsection • Intersex Surgery Subsection • Female Genital System Subsection • Maternity Care and Delivery Subsection • Endocrine System Subsection • Nervous System Subsection • Eye and Ocular Adnexa Subsection • Auditory System Subsection • Operating Microscope Subsection
Overview:	This chapter focuses on the CPT Surgery Male Genital System, Reproductive System Procedures, Intersex Surgery, Female Genital System, Maternity Care and Delivery, Endocrine System, Nervous System, Eye and Ocular Adnexa, Auditory System, and Operating Microscope subsections.
Objectives:	• Define key terms. • Explain the organization, format, and content of the CPT Male Genital System, Reproductive System Procedures, Intersex Surgery, Female Genital System, Maternity Care and Delivery, Endocrine System, Nervous System, Eye and Ocular Adnexa, Auditory System, and Operating Microscope subsections. • Interpret CPT surgery coding notes for the Male Genital System, Reproductive System Procedures, Intersex Surgery, Female Genital System, Maternity Care and Delivery, Endocrine System, Nervous System, Eye and Ocular Adnexa, Auditory System, and Operating Microscope subsections. • Assign CPT surgery codes from the Male Genital System, Reproductive System Procedures, Intersex Surgery, Female Genital System, Maternity Care and Delivery, Endocrine System, Nervous System, Eye and Ocular Adnexa, Auditory System, and Operating Microscope subsections. • Add CPT and/or HCPCS level II modifiers to codes as appropriate.

	Task	Resource
Prior to class:	• Read textbook and prepare lecture notes. • Review answers to chapter review. • Select workbook assignments for homework. • Prepare course syllabus. • Prepare chapter quiz.	• *3-2-1 Code It!*, Chapter 15 • *Instructor's Manual to Accompany 3-2-1 Code It!*, Chapter 15 • *Workbook to Accompany 3-2-1 Code It!*, Chapter 15 • *Instructor's Manual to Accompany 3-2-1 Code It!*, Introduction • *Instructor's Manual to Accompany 3-2-1 Code It!*, Chapter 15
Class # ___:	• Distribute and explain course syllabus. • Point out major features of textbook. • Review WebTutor™ features (if applicable). • Assign Chapter 15 as reading assignment. • Lecture on Chapter 15 content. • Encourage students to create flash cards. • Assign chapter review as homework.	• Prepared course syllabus • *3-2-1 Code It!*, Preface • *3-2-1 Code It!*, Preface • *3-2-1 Code It!*, Chapter 15 • Lecture notes prepared from *3-2-1 Code It!*, Chapter 15 • *3-2-1 Code It!*, Chapter 15 • *3-2-1 Code It!*, Chapter 15
Class # ___:	• Review previous class lecture and answer students' questions about chapter content. • Continue lecture on Chapter 15 content. • Collect homework (and grade). • Administer chapter quiz. • Assign Chapter 15 as reading assignment.	• Ask students to identify key topics and issues from previous class lecture. • *3-2-1 Code It!*, Chapter 15 • *Instructor's Manual to Accompany 3-2-1 Code It!*, Chapter 15 • *Instructor's Manual to Accompany 3-2-1 Code It!*, Chapter 15 • *3-2-1 Code It!*, Chapter 15
Lab # ___:	• Point out major features of workbook. • Communicate assignments to be accomplished during lab and explain how each is to be completed. • Rotate among students as they complete lab assignments to provide individual assistance. • Consider reviewing rough draft work during lab and allowing students to submit final draft at the beginning of the next lab class. • Assign additional workbook assignments for homework.	• *Workbook to Accompany 3-2-1 Code It!*, Preface • *Workbook to Accompany 3-2-1 Code It!*, Chapter 15
Assessment:	• Homework assignments • Chapter quiz • In-class participation • Lab assignments	

Chapter 16: CPT Radiology

Time:	• Instructor preparation (_____ hours) • In-class lecture (_____ hours) • In-class lab (if laboratory component is included as part of course) (_____ hours)
Topics:	• Radiology Terminology • Overview of Radiology Section • Radiology Section Guidelines • Radiology Subsections • Diagnostic Radiology (Diagnostic Imaging) • Diagnostic Ultrasound • Radiologic Guidance • Breast Mammography • Bone/Joint Studies • Radiation Oncology • Nuclear Medicine
Overview:	This chapter focuses on the CPT Radiology section, which includes diagnostic radiology (diagnostic imaging); diagnostic ultrasound; radiologic guidance; breast, mammography; bone/joint studies; radiation oncology; and nuclear medicine.
Objectives:	• Define key terms. • Explain the organization, format, and content of the CPT Radiology section. • Interpret CPT radiology coding guidelines and notes. • Assign CPT radiology codes. • Add CPT and/or HCPCS level II modifiers to codes as appropriate.

	Task	Resource
Prior to class:	• Read textbook and prepare lecture notes. • Review answers to chapter review. • Select workbook assignments for homework. • Prepare course syllabus. • Prepare chapter quiz.	• *3-2-1 Code It!*, Chapter 16 • *Instructor's Manual to Accompany 3-2-1 Code It!*, Chapter 16 • *Workbook to Accompany 3-2-1 Code It!*, Chapter 16 • *Instructor's Manual to Accompany 3-2-1 Code It!*, Introduction • *Instructor's Manual to Accompany 3-2-1 Code It!*, Chapter 16
Class # ____:	• Distribute and explain course syllabus. • Point out major features of textbook. • Review WebTutor™ features (if applicable). • Assign Chapter 16 as reading assignment. • Lecture on Chapter 16 content. • Encourage students to create flash cards. • Assign chapter review as homework.	• Prepared course syllabus • *3-2-1 Code It!*, Preface • *3-2-1 Code It!*, Preface • *3-2-1 Code It!*, Chapter 16 • Lecture notes prepared from *3-2-1 Code!*, Chapter 16 • *3-2-1 Code It!*, Chapter 16 • *3-2-1 Code It!*, Chapter 16
Class # ____:	• Review previous class lecture and answer students' questions about chapter content. • Continue lecture on Chapter 16 content. • Collect homework (and grade). • Administer chapter quiz. • Assign Chapter 16 as reading assignment.	• Ask students to identify key topics and issues from previous class lecture. • *3-2-1 Code It!*, Chapter 16 • *Instructor's Manual to Accompany 3-2-1 Code It!*, Chapter 16 • *Instructor's Manual to Accompany 3-2-1 Code It!*, Chapter 16 • *3-2-1 Code It!*, Chapter 16
Lab # ____:	• Point out major features of workbook. • Communicate assignments to be accomplished during lab and explain how each is to be completed. • Rotate among students as they complete lab assignments to provide individual assistance. • Consider reviewing rough draft work during lab and allowing students to submit final draft at the beginning of the next lab class. • Assign additional workbook assignments for homework.	• *Workbook to Accompany 3-2-1 Code It!*, Preface • *Workbook to Accompany 3-2-1 Code It!*, Chapter 16
Assessment:	• Homework assignments • Chapter quiz • In-class participation • Lab assignments	

Chapter 17: CPT Pathology and Laboratory

Time:	• Instructor preparation (_____ hours)
	• In-class lecture (_____ hours)
	• In-class lab (if laboratory component is included as part of course) (_____ hours)
Topics:	• Overview of Pathology and Laboratory Section
	• Pathology and Laboratory Section Guidelines
	• Pathology and Laboratory Subsections
Overview:	This chapter focuses on the CPT Pathology and Laboratory section.
Objectives:	• Define key terms.
	• Explain the organization, format, and content of the CPT Pathology and Laboratory section.
	• Interpret CPT pathology and laboratory coding guidelines and notes.
	• Assign CPT pathology and laboratory codes.
	• Add CPT and/or HCPCS level II modifiers to codes as appropriate.

	Task	Resource
Prior to class:	• Read textbook and prepare lecture notes.	• *3-2-1 Code It!*, Chapter 17
	• Review answers to chapter review.	• *Instructor's Manual to Accompany 3-2-1 Code It!*, Chapter 17
	• Select workbook assignments for homework.	• *Workbook to Accompany 3-2-1 Code It!*, Chapter 17
	• Prepare course syllabus.	• *Instructor's Manual to Accompany 3-2-1 Code It!*, Introduction
	• Prepare chapter quiz.	• *Instructor's Manual to Accompany 3-2-1 Code It!*, Chapter 17
Class # ___:	• Distribute and explain course syllabus.	• Prepared course syllabus
	• Point out major features of textbook.	• *3-2-1 Code It!*, Preface
	• Review WebTutor™ features (if applicable).	• *3-2-1 Code It!*, Preface
	• Assign Chapter 17 as reading assignment.	• *3-2-1 Code It!*, Chapter 17
	• Lecture on Chapter 17 content.	• Lecture notes prepared from *3-2-1 Code!*, Chapter 17
	• Encourage students to create flash cards.	• *3-2-1 Code It!*, Chapter 17
	• Assign chapter review as homework.	• *3-2-1 Code It!*, Chapter 17
Class # ___:	• Review previous class lecture and answer students' questions about chapter content.	• Ask students to identify key topics and issues from previous class lecture.
	• Continue lecture on Chapter 17 content.	• *3-2-1 Code It!*, Chapter 17
	• Collect homework (and grade).	• *Instructor's Manual to Accompany 3-2-1 Code It!*, Chapter 17
	• Administer chapter quiz.	• *Instructor's Manual to Accompany 3-2-1 Code It!*, Chapter 17
	• Assign Chapter 17 as reading assignment.	• *3-2-1 Code It!*, Chapter 17
Lab # ___:	• Point out major features of workbook.	• *Workbook to Accompany 3-2-1 Code It!*, Preface
	• Communicate assignments to be accomplished during lab and explain how each is to be completed.	• *Workbook to Accompany 3-2-1 Code It!*, Chapter 17
	• Rotate among students as they complete lab assignments to provide individual assistance.	
	• Consider reviewing rough draft work during lab and allowing students to submit final draft at the beginning of the next lab class.	
	• Assign additional workbook assignments for homework.	
Assessment:	• Homework assignments	
	• Chapter quiz	
	• In-class participation	
	• Lab assignments	

Chapter 18: CPT Medicine

Time:	• Instructor preparation (_____ hours) • In-class lecture (_____ hours) • In-class lab (if laboratory component is included as part of course) (_____ hours)
Topics:	• Overview of Medicine Section • Medicine Section Guidelines • Medicine Subsections
Overview:	This chapter focuses on the CPT Medicine section.
Objectives:	• Define key terms. • Explain the organization, format, and content of the CPT Medicine section. • Interpret CPT medicine coding guidelines and notes. • Assign CPT medicine codes. • Add CPT and/or HCPCS level II modifiers to codes as appropriate.

	Task	Resource
Prior to class:	• Read textbook and prepare lecture notes. • Review answers to chapter review. • Select workbook assignments for homework. • Prepare course syllabus. • Prepare chapter quiz.	• *3-2-1 Code It!*, Chapter 18 • *Instructor's Manual to Accompany 3-2-1 Code It!*, Chapter 18 • *Workbook to Accompany 3-2-1 Code It!*, Chapter 18 • *Instructor's Manual to Accompany 3-2-1 Code It!*, Introduction • *Instructor's Manual to Accompany 3-2-1 Code It!*, Chapter 18
Class # ___:	• Distribute and explain course syllabus. • Point out major features of textbook. • Review WebTutor™ features (if applicable). • Assign Chapter 18 as reading assignment. • Lecture on Chapter 18 content. • Encourage students to create flash cards. • Assign chapter review as homework.	• Prepared course syllabus • *3-2-1 Code It!*, Preface • *3-2-1 Code It!*, Preface • *3-2-1 Code It!*, Chapter 18 • Lecture notes prepared from *3-2-1 Code!*, Chapter 18 • *3-2-1 Code It!*, Chapter 18 • *3-2-1 Code It!*, Chapter 18
Class # ___:	• Review previous class lecture and answer students' questions about chapter content. • Continue lecture on Chapter 18 content. • Collect homework (and grade). • Administer chapter quiz. • Assign Chapter 18 as reading assignment.	• Ask students to identify key topics and issues from previous class lecture. • *3-2-1 Code It!*, Chapter 18 • *Instructor's Manual to Accompany 3-2-1 Code It!*, Chapter 18 • *Instructor's Manual to Accompany 3-2-1 Code It!*, Chapter 18 • *3-2-1 Code It!*, Chapter 18
Lab # ___:	• Point out major features of workbook. • Communicate assignments to be accomplished during lab and explain how each is to be completed. • Rotate among students as they complete lab assignments to provide individual assistance. • Consider reviewing rough draft work during lab and allowing students to submit final draft at the beginning of the next lab class. • Assign additional workbook assignments for homework.	• *Workbook to Accompany 3-2-1 Code It!*, Preface • *Workbook to Accompany 3-2-1 Code It!*, Chapter 18
Assessment:	• Homework assignments • Chapter quiz • In-class participation • Lab assignments	

Chapter 19: Insurance and Reimbursement

Time:	• Instructor preparation (_____ hours) • In-class lecture (_____ hours) • In-class lab (if laboratory component is included as part of course) (_____ hours)
Topics:	• Third-Party Payers • Health Care Reimbursement Systems • Impact of HIPAA on Reimbursement
Overview:	This chapter focuses on health care insurance and reimbursement issues, including third-party payers, health care reimbursement systems, and the impact of the Health Insurance Portability and Accountability Act of 1996 on reimbursement.
Objectives:	• Define key terms. • Identify and provide examples of third-party payers. • Describe Medicare prospective payment systems (PPS) and fee schedules. • State the function of a chargemaster review. • Delineate the regulatory provisions of the Health Insurance Portability and Accountability Act of 1996 (HIPAA).

	Task	Resource
Prior to class:	• Read textbook and prepare lecture notes. • Review answers to chapter review. • Select workbook assignments for homework. • Prepare course syllabus. • Prepare chapter quiz.	• *3-2-1 Code It!*, Chapter 19 • *Instructor's Manual to Accompany 3-2-1 Code It!*, Chapter 19 • *Workbook to Accompany 3-2-1 Code It!*, Chapter 19 • *Instructor's Manual to Accompany 3-2-1 Code It!*, Introduction • *Instructor's Manual to Accompany 3-2-1 Code It!*, Chapter 19
Class # ___:	• Distribute and explain course syllabus. • Point out major features of textbook. • Review WebTutor™ features (if applicable). • Assign Chapter 19 as reading assignment. • Lecture on Chapter 19 content. • Encourage students to create flash cards. • Assign chapter review as homework.	• Prepared course syllabus • *3-2-1 Code It!*, Preface • *3-2-1 Code It!*, Preface • *3-2-1 Code It!*, Chapter 19 • Lecture notes prepared from *3-2-1 Code!*, Chapter 19 • *3-2-1 Code It!*, Chapter 19 • *3-2-1 Code It!*, Chapter 19
Class # ___:	• Review previous class lecture and answer students' questions about chapter content. • Continue lecture on Chapter 19 content. • Collect homework (and grade). • Administer chapter quiz. • Assign Chapter 19 as reading assignment.	• Ask students to identify key topics and issues from previous class lecture. • *3-2-1 Code It!*, Chapter 19 • *Instructor's Manual to Accompany 3-2-1 Code It!*, Chapter 19 • *Instructor's Manual to Accompany 3-2-1 Code It!*, Chapter 19 • *3-2-1 Code It!*, Chapter 19
Lab # ___:	• Point out major features of workbook. • Communicate assignments to be accomplished during lab and explain how each is to be completed. • Rotate among students as they complete lab assignments to provide individual assistance. • Consider reviewing rough draft work during lab and allowing students to submit final draft at the beginning of the next lab class. • Assign additional workbook assignments for homework.	• *Workbook to Accompany 3-2-1 Code It!*, Preface • *Workbook to Accompany 3-2-1 Code It!*, Chapter 19
Assessment:	• Homework assignments • Chapter quiz • In-class participation • Lab assignments	

Answer Keys to Chapter Exercises and Reviews

Chapter 1
Overview of Coding

EXERCISE 1.1 – CAREER AS A CODER

1. c
2. a
3. b
4. c
5. b
6. c
7. e
8. a
9. b
10. d

EXERCISE 1.2 – PROFESSIONAL ASSOCIATIONS AND DISCUSSION BOARDS

1. c
2. a
3. b
4. a
5. c

EXERCISE 1.3 – OVERVIEW OF CODING

1. b
2. a
3. a
4. a
5. a
6. b
7. b
8. a
9. a
10. b

EXERCISE 1.4 – DOCUMENTATION AS THE BASIS FOR CODING

1. a
2. b
3. b
4. b
5. b
6. medical record
7. demographic data
8. continuity of care
9. medical necessity
10. manual
11. source-oriented
12. integrated
13. electronic medical record (EMR)
14. optical disk imaging (or document imaging)
15. jukebox

EXERCISE 1.5 – HEALTH DATA COLLECTION

1. medical management
2. case abstracting
3. CMS-1500
4. UB-04 (or CMS-1450)
5. medical necessity

REVIEW

Multiple Choice

1. a	8. d	15. b
2. d	9. a	16. d
3. c	10. a	17. b
4. b	11. c	18. a
5. b	12. a	19. b
6. c	13. c	20. c
7. c	14. b	

Chapter 2
Introduction to ICD-9-CM Coding

EXERCISE 2.1 – OVERVIEW OF ICD-9-CM

1. 1979
2. three
3. National Center for Health Statistics (NCHS); Centers for Medicare & Medicaid Services (CMS)
4. Medicare Prescription Drug, Improvement, and Modernization Act (MMA)
5. subscription
6. encoder
7. Medicare Catastrophic Coverage Act of 1988
8. medical necessity
9. chest pain
10. multiple lacerations

EXERCISE 2.2 – ICD-9-CM TABULAR LIST OF DISEASES

1. Tabular List of Diseases
2. Diagnostic and Statistical Manual of Mental Disorders (DSM)
3. V codes
4. E codes
5. Morphology of Neoplasms (M codes)
6. neoplasms
7. benign; malignant
8. Classification of Drugs by AHFS List
9. Classification of Industrial Accidents According to Agency
10. List of Three-Digit Categories

EXERCISE 2.3 – ICD-9-CM INDEX TO DISEASES

1. Index to Diseases
2. Table of Drugs and Chemicals
3. letter-by-letter
4. Launois-Cleret syndrome
5. numerical
6. boldfaced
7. nonessential modifiers

8. essential modifiers
9. Asthmatic
10. History

> ## Note:
> The main term is History in the Index to Diseases. The diagnosis "history of affective psychosis" indicates that the patient no longer has the condition. Therefore, do not refer to main term Psychosis and subterm affective, which would result in an incorrect code assignment.

11. 5	15. 1	19. 7
12. 2	16. 9	20. 3
13. 6	17. 8	
14. 4	18. 10	

> ## Note:
> H disease is sequenced after Hb because it is interpreted as "Hdisease" according to letter-by-letter alphabetization rules, which means that spaces and hyphens are ignored.

EXERCISE 2.4 – ICD-9-CM TABULAR LIST OF PROCEDURES AND INDEX TO PROCEDURES

1. Tabular List of Procedures and Index to Procedures
2. *Current Procedural Terminology* (CPT); *Healthcare Financing Administration Common Procedure Coding System, Level II (national)*
3. December 31, 2003
4. two
5. 17

EXERCISE 2.5 – OFFICIAL GUIDELINES FOR CODING AND REPORTING

1. cooperating parties for the ICD-9-CM
2. AHA; AHIMA; CMS; NCHS
3. HIPAA
4. encounter
5. provider

REVIEW

Multiple Choice

1. a	5. c	9. c
2. b	6. a	10. d
3. a	7. b	
4. c	8. a	

Matching

11. b   13. a   15. e

12. c   14. d

Coding Practice

ICD-9-CM Index to Diseases and Tabular List of Diseases

553.20   16. Abdominal <u>hernia</u>

790.29   17. <u>Abnormal</u> nonfasting glucose tolerance test

382.9   18. Acute <u>otitis</u> media

621.30   19. <u>Hyperplasia</u> of endometrium

818.0   20. Broken arm (<u>Fracture</u>)

Note:

The see *instruction that appears next to main term* Broken, *subterm* bone *directs the coder to go to main term* Fracture, *by site.* Subterm *arm (closed)* is selected because the condition does not document an "open" fracture, *which involves a fractured bone and* an open wound of adjacent or overlying soft tissues at the site of the fracture.

748.4   21. Congenital fibrocystic <u>disease</u> of the lung (<u>Fibrocystic, disease</u>)

Note:

The see also *instruction that appears next to* Disease, fibrocystic *refers to the coder to main term* Fibrocystic, disease *because the original main term does not classify the condition.*

715.90   22. Degenerative <u>arthritis</u>

610.1   23. Fibrocystic <u>disease</u> of breasts

448.0   24. Hereditary <u>epistaxis</u>

V10.9   25. <u>History</u> of cancer

Note:

Cancer *is not listed as a subterm below* History (personal) *of. Therefore, refer to subterm* maliganant (of) NEC *to assign V16.9. (You also don't know what type of cancer was present.)*

ICD-9-CM Index to Procedures and Tabular List of Procedures

40.11	26. Biopsy, axillary lymph node
51.23	27. Laparoscopic cholecystectomy
57.21	28. Cystoscopy
54.11	29. Exploratory laparotomy
87.73	30. Intravenous pyelogram
47.19	31. Incidental appendectomy
22.12	32. Open biopsy of nasal sinus
60.11	33. Percutaneous biopsy of prostate
01.24	34. Right frontal craniotomy
57.33	35. Transurethral biopsy of bladder

Chapter 3
ICD-9-CM Coding Conventions

EXERCISE 3.1 – FORMAT

487.8	1. Gastric influenza
701.1	2. Acquired pilaris pityriasis
V52.1	3. Admission for adjustment of artificial leg
309.24	4. Adjustment reaction with anxious mood
307.1	5. Voluntary starvation
38.07	6. Abdominal venotomy
51.24	7. Laparoscopic cholecystectomy, partial
47.11	8. Incidental laparoscopic appendectomy
14.73	9. Vitrectomy, anterior approach
85.12	10. Open breast biopsy

EXERCISE 3.2 – EPONYMS

524.60	1. Costen syndrome or complex
755.54	2. Madelung's deformity
362.12	3. Coat disease
716.00	4. Kaschin-Beck disease
386.00	5. Meniere disease
082.1	6. Mediterranean tick fever
22.39	7. Caldwell-Luc operation
81.44	8. Roux-Goldthwait operation
89.42	9. Masters two-step stress test
59.4	10. Millin-Read operation

EXERCISE 3.3 – ABBREVIATIONS

287.2	1. Purpura
553.00	2. Femoral hernia
410.10	3. Anterior wall myocardial infarction
041.89	4. Bacillus infection
871.4	5. Laceration of the eyeball
781.0	6. Tremor
62.41	7. Bilateral orchidectomy
84.24	8. Upper arm reattachment

96.56   9. Irrigation of the bronchus

23.19   10. Surgical removal of a tooth

EXERCISE 3.4 – PUNCTUATION

046.19, 294.11   1. Spastic pseudosclerosis with dementia and behavioral disturbances

084.9, 573.2   2. Malaria with hepatitis

030.3   3. Dimorphous leprosy

00.66   4. Percutaneous transluminal coronary angioplasty

245.0   5. Acute pyogenic thyroiditis

01.09   6. Cranial puncture, subdural tap

733.09   7. Preiser disease

243   8. Cretinism

68.23   9. Endometrial ablation

24.5   10. Alveoloplasty

EXERCISE 3.5 – BOXED NOTES

853.01   1. Traumatic brain hemorrhage with no loss of consciousness

884.0   2. Multiple open wounds to arms

296.21   3. Single episode of mild involutional affective psychosis

730.16   4. Chronic periostitis with osteomyelitis of the lower leg

533.40   5. Recurrent bleeding peptic ulcer

919.3   6. Infected blister

216.7   7. Cellular blue nevus on calf (Neoplasm Table, skin, benign)

91.35   8. Toxicology examination of urine specimen

81.02   9. Anterior spinal fusion of C4-C6

81.62

54.51   10. Laparoscopic lysis of abdominal adhesions

EXERCISE 3.6 – TABLES

405.11   1. Benign hypertension due to renal stenosis (Hypertension Table)

405.99   2. Secondary hypertension (Hypertension Table)

401.0   3. Malignant idiopathic hypertension (Hypertension Table)

239.1   4. Ethmoid tumor (Neoplasm Table)

173.3   5. Basal cell carcinoma, skin of external cheek (Neoplasm Table)

155.2   6. Carcinoma of the liver (Neoplasm Table)

185   7. Prostate cancer (Neoplasm Table)

987.8, E982.8, E849.9   8. Poisoning due to inhalation of paint fumes (Table of Drugs and Chemicals)

785.59, E943.3   9. Circulatory collapse due to therapeutic use of magnesium sulfate (Table of Drugs and Chemicals)

969.0, E854.0, E849.9   10. Accidental overdose of antidepressants (Table of Drugs and Chemicals)

EXERCISE 3.7 – INCLUDES NOTES

323.9	1. Meningoencephalitis
403.90	2. Nephrosclerosis
534.90	3. Anastomotic ulcer
401.9	4. Hypertensive vascular degeneration
682.9	5. Lymphangitis, acute
72.71	6. Malstrom's vacuum extraction with episiotomy
76.70	7. Reduction and fixation of facial fracture
81.00	8. Arthrodesis of spine with internal fixation
88.68	9. Impedance phlebography with venipuncture for injection of contrast material
14.39	10. Repair of retinal defect

EXERCISE 3.8 – EXCLUDES NOTES

429.2	1. Cardiovascular disease
447.6	2. Arteritis
626.0	3. Absence of menstruation
694.0	4. Herpetiformis dermatosis
746.87	5. Dextrocardia
780.4	6. Vertigo
896.2	7. Traumatic amputation of feet
190.1	8. Malignant neoplasm of eye orbit
251.2	9. Hypoglycemia
333.83	10. Spasmotic torticollis

EXERCISE 3.9 – INCLUSION TERMS

006.1	1. Chronic amebic dysentery
116.0	2. Chicago disease
207.20	3. Thrombocytic leukemia
330.1	4. Tay-Sachs disease
590.2	5. Carbuncle of kidney
21.31	6. Nasal polypectomy
36.39	7. Intrapericardial poudrage
75.38	8. Transcervical fetal oxygen saturation monitoring (intrapartum)
92.04	9. Radio-cobalt B12 Schilling test
68.31	10. Classic infrafascial SEMM hysterectomy (abdominal)

EXERCISE 3.10 – OTHER, OTHER SPECIFIED, AND UNSPECIFIED CODES

543.9	1. Appendicular fistula
633.90	2. Ectopic pregnancy
674.84	3. Hepatorenal syndrome following delivery (postpartum condition)
445.89	4. Arterial atheroembolism

361.9	5. Detached retina
996.79	6. Complications due to eye implant
87.59	7. Cholecystogram
93.96	8. Oxygen by nasal cannula
47.09	9. Abdominal appendectomy
23.19	10. Removal of impacted tooth

EXERCISE 3.11 – ETIOLOGY AND MANIFESTATION RULES

252.1, 366.42	1. Tetanic cataract in hypoparathyroidism
135, 425.8	2. Cardiac sarcoidosis
017.00	3. Tuberculosis of the eyelid
585.9, 420.0	4. Uremia with pericarditis
090.0, 567.0	5. Congenital syphilitic peritonitits
250.50, 362.02	6. Diabetic proliferative retinopathy
002.0, 730.80	7. Osteomyelitis due to typhoid
710.0, 424.91	8. Verrucous endocarditis
390, 517.1	9. Rheumatic pneumonia
015.10, 727.01	10. Synovitis of the hip in tuberculosis

EXERCISE 3.12 – AND

099.52	1. Venereal disease of the rectum due to Chlamydia
170.3	2. Malignant neoplasm of costal cartilage
253.0	3. Acromegaly
516.9	4. Parietoalveolar pneumopathy
232.4	5. Carcinoma in situ of scalp
528.3	6. Abscess, mouth
732.1	7. Juvenile osteochondrosis, head of femur
767.0	8. Subdural hemorrhage during birth
82.11	9. Tenotomy of hand
81.06	10. Lumbar fusion, anterior technique

EXERCISE 3.13 – DUE TO

696.0	1. Arthritis due to psoriasis
440.21	2. Angiosclerotica intermittens dysbasia due to atherosclerosis
277.00	3. Cirrhosis due to cystic fibrosis
099.0	4. Bubo due to Hemophilus ducreyi
286.7	5. Coagulation factor deficiency due to liver disease
244.1	6. Hypothyroidism due to radioactive iodine
252.01, 737.42	7. Lordosis due to fibrosa cystica osteitis

478.75 _____   8. Airway <u>obstruction</u> due to laryngospasm

690.10, 380.13   9. <u>Otitis</u> externa due to seborrheic dermatitis

477.1 _____   10. Allergic <u>rhinitis</u> due to food allergy

EXERCISE 3.14 – IN

153.9 _____   1. <u>Adenocarcinoma</u> in adenomatous polyposis coli

308.0 _____   2. <u>Anxiety</u> in acute stress reaction

E974 _____   3. Bayonet <u>wound</u> during legal intervention

671.04 _____   4. <u>Varicose</u> vein as postpartum condition

052.7, 370.44   5. <u>Keratoconjunctivitis</u> in chickenpox

378.20 _____   6. <u>Strabismus</u> in intermittent neuromuscular disorder

290.20 _____   7. Paranoid <u>state</u> in senile brain disease

115.92 _____   8. Focal <u>retinochoroiditis</u> in histoplasmosis

660.20 _____   9. <u>Rectocele</u> in pregnancy causing obstructed labor

078.6 _____   10. <u>Nephrosis</u> in epidemic hemorrhagic fever

EXERCISE 3.15 – WITH

540.0 _____   1. <u>Appendicitis</u> with perforation

242.10 _____   2. <u>Thyrotoxicosis</u> with uninodular adenomatous goiter

860.3 _____   3. Traumatic <u>hemothorax</u> with open wound into thorax

314.01 _____   4. Attention deficit <u>disorder</u> with hyperactivity

740.0 _____   5. Skull <u>agenesis</u> with anencephalus

35.61 _____   6. <u>Closure</u> of foramen ovale with tissue graft

38.34 _____   7. <u>Correction</u> of coarctation of aorta with anastomosis

66.39 _____   8. <u>Destruction</u> of fallopian tube with ligation

15.6 _____   9. Extraocular muscle <u>operation</u> with revision

02.94 _____   10. <u>Removal</u> of halo traction with synchronous replacement

EXERCISE 3.16 – CROSS-REFERENCES

637.30 _____   1. <u>Uremia</u> with abortion

799.89 _____   2. <u>Toxicosis</u>

551.8 _____   3. <u>Strangulated</u> gangrenous abdominal hernia

755.59 _____   4. <u>Undescended</u> arm

788.69 _____   5. <u>Urinary</u> abnormality

88.32 _____   6. Contrast <u>x-ray</u> of ankle

39.59 _____   7. <u>Plasty</u> of peripheral blood vessel

38.10 _____   8. <u>Removal</u> of thrombus with endarterectomy

78.90, 79.00   9. Fracture <u>repair</u> with insertion of bone growth stimulator

53.00 _____   10. Halsted <u>operation</u>

REVIEW

Matching I

1. d
2. c
3. e
4. a
5. b

Matching II

6. e
7. c
8. b
9. d
10. a

Multiple Choice

11. d
12. d
13. b
14. b
15. a
16. c
17. a
18. d
19. c
20. c
21. b
22. c
23. b
24. b
25. c
26. d
27. a
28. b
29. a
30. d

Chapter 4
ICD-9-CM Coding Guidelines

EXERCISE 4.1 – ICD-9-CM OFFICIAL GUIDELINES FOR CODING AND REPORTING

1. cooperating parties for the ICD-9-CM
2. encounter
3. provider
4. HIPAA
5. structure and conventions
6. principal diagnosis
7. additional diagnoses
8. comorbidities and complications
9. outpatient coding and reporting
10. present on admission (POA) reporting guidelines

EXERCISE 4.2 – GENERAL ICD-9-CM DIAGNOSIS CODING GUIDELINES

1. F

> **Note:**
>
> *The boxed note below the entry indicates that a fifth-digit subclassification is required for category 948 codes.*

2. F

> **Note:**
>
> *Always verify codes in the Tabular List of Diseases.*

3. T   4. T   5. F

> **Note:**
>
> *When established diagnoses are coded, do not assign codes to associated signs and symptoms.*

6. T   7. F

> **Note:**
>
> When signs and symptoms are integral to the disease process, they are included in the code for the established or definitive disease.

8. T   9. T   10. F

> **Note:**
>
> When possible, assign separate codes for the acute (or subacute) and chronic conditions. (Sometimes there is a combination code for acute and chronic conditions.)

11. F

> **Note:**
>
> Multiple coding involves assigning two or more codes to completely classify the elements of a complex diagnostic statement, which contain words or phrases such as due to, incidental to, secondary to, with, or other similar terminology.

12. T   13. T   14. F

> **Note:**
>
> There is no time limit on when a late effect residual code can be reported.

15. F

> **Note:**
>
> Code any condition described at the time of encounter/visit as "impending" or "threatened" as follows: If the condition did occur, code as confirmed diagnosis; if the condition did not occur, reference the Index to Diseases to determine if the condition has a subentry term for "impending" or "threatened" and reference main term entries for "Impending" and "Threatened"; if subterms impending or threatened are listed, assign the code; and if subterms impending or threatened are not listed, code the existing underlying condition(s), not the condition described as "impending" or "threatened."

EXERCISE 4.3 – GENERAL ICD-9-CM PROCEDURE CODING GUIDELINES

1. F

> **Note:**
>
> The ICD-9-CM procedure classification is published in Volume 3, and it includes both an Index to Procedures and a Tabular List of Procedures.

2. F

> **Note:**
>
> The coding conventions that appear in the ICD-9-CM Index to Procedures and Tabular List of Procedures are similar to those used in the Index to Diseases, Index to External Causes and Injuries, and Tabular List of Diseases.

3. T   4. F

> **Note:**
>
> Index to Procedures main terms are organized in alphabetical order according to type of procedure, common name of the procedure, and eponyms.

5. T   6. T   7. F

> **Note:**
>
> Modifiers are not assigned to ICD-9-CM codes. (They are assigned to CPT codes.)

8. F

> **Note:**
>
> The phrase —omit code is located after an Index to Procedures main term or subterm, and it means that the coder should not assign the code because it is considered an integral part of the procedure.

9. F

> **Note:**
>
> A combination code is a single code assigned to classify two or more procedures.

10. T

85.50	11. Augmentation mammoplasty (or Augmentation mammoplasty)
41.32	12. Closed aspiration biopsy of spleen
05.32	13. Injection of neurolytic agent into sympathetic nerve
65.41	14. Laparoscopic unilateral salpingo-oophorectomy
38.59	15. Ligation and stripping of varicose veins, left leg
60.12	16. Open biopsy of prostate
42.21	17. Operative esophagoscopy (by incision)
06.81	18. Parathyroidectomy, complete
72.51	19. Partial breech extraction with forceps to head
81.52	20. Partial hip replacement

55.04	21. Percutaneous <u>nephrostomy</u> with fragmentation
22.01	22. <u>Puncture</u> of nasal sinus for aspiration
00.54	23. <u>Replacement</u> of only cardiac resynchronization defibrillator pulse, generator device
11.31	24. <u>Transposition</u> of pterygium
19.52	25. Type II <u>tympanoplasty</u>

EXERCISE 4.4 – ICD-9-CM CHAPTER 1 – INFECTIOUS AND PARASITIC DISEASES (001–139)

042	1. <u>AIDS</u>
005.1	2. <u>Botulism</u>
088.81	3. <u>Lyme</u> disease
055.1	4. Postmeasles <u>pneumonia</u>
071	5. <u>Rabies</u>

EXERCISE 4.5 – ICD-9-CM CHAPTER 2 – NEOPLASMS (140–239)

233.1	1. Carcinoma in situ, cervix uteri (<u>neoplasm</u>)

> **Note:**
>
> *In the ICD-9-CM index, go to the Neoplasm Table, locate main term Cervix and locate code 233.1 in the Carcinoma in situ column.*

181	2. <u>Choriocarcinoma</u> (female patient)

> **Note:**
>
> *In the ICD-9-CM index, locate main term Choriocarcinoma, subterm unspecified site, and 2nd qualifier female.*

228.00	3. <u>Hemangioma</u>
176.9	4. <u>Kaposi</u> sarcoma
214.1	5. <u>Lipoma</u>, skin of abdomen

EXERCISE 4.6 – CHAPTER 3 – ENDOCRINE, NUTRITIONAL AND METABOLIC DISEASES, AND IMMUNITY DISORDERS (240–279)

250.03	1. <u>Diabetes mellitus</u>, type 1 uncontrolled
250.00	2. <u>Diabetes mellitus</u>, type 2
253.1	3. Forbes-Albright <u>syndrome</u>
278.01	4. Morbid <u>obesity</u>
256.4	5. <u>Polycystic</u> ovaries

EXERCISE 4.7 – CHAPTER 4 – DISEASES OF THE BLOOD AND BLOOD-FORMING ORGANS (280–289)

289.0	1. Acquired <u>polycythemia</u>
285.1	2. Acute posthemorrhagic <u>anemia</u>
288.09	3. <u>Agranuloycytosis</u>
281.9	4. Chronic <u>anemia</u>

> **Note:**
>
> *Locate code 281.9 by referring to main term* Anemia *and subterm* chronic simple. *Do not assign code 285.9 for "chronic anemia."*

289.51	5. Chronic congestive <u>splenomegaly</u>

EXERCISE 4.8 – CHAPTER 5 – MENTAL DISORDERS (290–319)

331.0	1. <u>Alzheimer's</u> disease
295.32	2. Chronic paranoid <u>schizophrenia</u>
291.0	3. <u>Delirium</u> tremens
305.62	4. Episodic cocaine <u>abuse</u>
296.30	5. Major depressive <u>disorder</u>, recurrent episode

EXERCISE 4.9 – CHAPTER 6 – DISEASES OF THE NERVOUS SYSTEM AND SENSE ORGANS (320–389)

380.12	1. Acute <u>swimmers'</u> ear
351.0	2. <u>Bell</u> palsy
368.2	3. <u>Diplopia</u>
343.2	4. Infantile <u>quadriplegia</u>
324.1	5. Intraspinal <u>abscess</u>

EXERCISE 4.10 – CHAPTER 7 – DISEASES OF THE CIRCULATORY SYSTEM (390–459)

410.21	1. Acute myocardial <u>infarction,</u> inferolateral wall, initial episode of care
391.1	2. Acute rheumatic <u>endocarditis</u>
438.11	3. <u>Aphasia, late</u> effect of cerebrovascular disease
401.1	4. Benign <u>hypertension</u>
396.3	5. Mitral and aortic valve <u>insufficiency</u>

EXERCISE 4.11 – CHAPTER 8 - DISEASES OF THE RESPIRATORY SYSTEM (460–519)

461.1	1. Acute frontal <u>sinusitis</u>
477.0	2. Allergic <u>rhinitis</u> due to pollen
518.0	3. <u>Atelectasis</u>

496____   4. Chronic obstructive pulmonary <u>disease</u>
464.4   5. <u>Croup</u>

EXERCISE 4.12 – CHAPTER 9 – DISEASES OF THE DIGESTIVE SYSTEM (520–579)

534.11   1. Acute gastrojejunal <u>ulcer</u>, with perforation and obstruction
528.2____   2. <u>Canker</u> sore
555.9____   3. Crohn <u>disease</u>
530.81   4. Gastroesophageal <u>reflux</u>
550.90   5. Inguinal <u>hernia</u>

EXERCISE 4.13 – CHAPTER 10 – DISEASES OF THE GENITOURINARY SYSTEM (580–629)

604.0   1. <u>Abscess</u> of epididymis
610.1   2. Chronic cystic <u>mastitis</u>
601.1   3. Chronic <u>prostatitis</u>
596.3   4. <u>Diverticulitis</u> of bladder
626.2   5. Excessive <u>menstruation</u>

EXERCISE 4.14 – CHAPTER 11 – COMPLICATIONS OF PREGNANCY, CHILDBIRTH, AND THE PUERPERIUM (630–677)

658.40   1. <u>Amnionitis</u>
676.24   2. <u>Engorgement</u> of breasts (postpartum)
642.33   3. Gestational <u>hypertension</u> (antepartum)

> **Note:**
>
> In the ICD-9-CM Index to Diseases, go to the hypertension table and locate subterm complicating pregnancy and 2nd qualifier gestational.

661.41   4. Incoordinate uterine <u>contractions</u>, delivered
665.34   5. <u>Laceration</u> of cervix (postpartum complication)

> **Note:**
>
> Do not assign code 622.3, which classifies an "old laceration of cervix."

EXERCISE 4.15 – CHAPTER 12 – DISEASES OF THE SKIN AND SUBCUTANEOUS TISSUE (680–709)

704.01   1. <u>Alopecia</u> areata
680.6____   2. <u>Carbuncle</u>, left ankle
707.00   3. Decubitus <u>ulcer</u>

| 684 | 4. Impetigo |
| 701.4 | 5. Keloid |

EXERCISE 4.16 – CHAPTER 13 – DISEASES OF THE MUSCULOSKELETAL AND CONNECTIVE TISSUE (710–739)

| 719.49 | 1. Arthralgia, hand, lower leg, and ankle |

> **Note:**
>
> Assign code 719.49 for "multiple sites." Do not assign separate codes 719.44, 719.46, and 719.47 when a combination code for "multiple sites" is available.

735.5	2. Claw toe (acquired)
718.45	3. Contracture of joint, pelvic region
721.5	4. Kissing spine
728.85	5. Muscle spasm

EXERCISE 4.17 – CHAPTER 14 – CONGENITAL ANOMALIES (740–759)

747.21	1. Anomalies of aortic arch
746.86	2. Congenital heart block
742.3	3. Congenital hydrocephalus
743.03	4. Cystic eyeball, congenital
750.13	5. Fissure of tongue, congenital

> **Note:**
>
> Do not assign code 529.5, which is an acquired condition. For congenital "fissure of tongue," assign code 750.13.

EXERCISE 4.18 – CHAPTER 15 – CERTAIN CONDITIONS ORIGINATING IN THE PERINATAL PERIOD (760–779)

770.83	1. Cyanotic attacks of newborn
766.0	2. Exceptionally large baby
767.5	3. Facial palsy, newborn
779.3	4. Feeding problems in newborn
772.0	5. Fetal blood loss

EXERCISE 4.19 – CHAPTER 16 – SIGNS, SYMPTOMS, AND ILL-DEFINED CONDITIONS (780–799)

796.1	1. Abnormal reflex
781.3	2. Ataxia
790.93	3. Elevated prostate specific antigen

783.41   4. <u>Failure</u> to thrive (child)

780.51   5. <u>Insomnia</u> with sleep apnea

EXERCISE 4.20 – CHAPTER 17 – INJURY AND POISONING (800–999)

802.22	1. Closed <u>fracture</u> mandible, subcondylar
831.04	2. Closed <u>dislocation</u> of clavicle
850.11	3. <u>Concussion</u> with brief loss of consciousness (30 minutes)
945.22	4. Foot <u>burn</u>, blisters, epidermal loss (second-degree)
861.02	5. Heart <u>laceration</u> without penetration of heart chambers
708.0, E930.0	6. <u>Hives</u> resulting from <u>penicillin</u> taken as prescribed
967.0, 780.01, E950.1	7. <u>Coma</u> due to <u>overdose of barbiturates</u> (attempted <u>suicide</u>)
995.20, E948.6	8. <u>Adverse reaction</u> to <u>pertussis vaccine</u>

> **Note:**
>
> The adverse reaction is not stated. Therefore, assign code 995.20.

971.2, 980.0, E855.5, E860.0, 427.9   9. <u>Cardiac arrhythmia</u> due to <u>interaction of prescribed ephedrine and alcohol intoxication</u> (<u>accident</u>)

> **Note:**
>
> Do not assign code E941.2 as an adverse effect external cause because combining the prescribed drug with alcohol makes this a poisoning case.

963.0, 780.09, E858.1   10. <u>Stupor</u> due to <u>overdose of Nytol</u> (<u>accident</u>)

EXERCISE 4.21 – SUPPLEMENTARY CLASSIFICATION OF FACTORS INFLUENCING HEALTH STATUS AND CONTACT WITH HEALTH SERVICES (V01–V84)

V59.3	1. Bone marrow <u>donor</u>
V58.11	2. <u>Chemotherapy</u> encounter
V70.3	3. <u>Examination</u> for summer camp
V01.3	4. <u>Exposure</u> to smallpox
V17.1	5. Family <u>history</u> of stroke

EXERCISE 4.22 – SUPPLEMENTAL CLASSIFICATION OF EXTERNAL CAUSES OF INJURY AND POISONING (E800–E999)

E853.2   1. Accidental poisoning of diazepam (<u>Table of Drugs and Chemicals</u>)

> **Note:**
>
> In the ICD-9-CM Index to Diseases, go to the Table of Drugs and Chemicals, locate main term Diazepam, and locate the code in the Accidental column.

E898.0	2. <u>Burning</u> bedclothes
E837.9	3. <u>Explosion</u> in watercraft
E881.0	4. <u>Fall</u> from ladder
E849.4	5. Foot injury taking place on baseball field (<u>accident</u>)

> **Note:**
>
> *In the ICD-9-CM Index to External Causes and Injuries, go to main term* Accident *and locate subterm* occurring (at) (in) *and 2nd qualifier* baseball field.

REVIEW

Multiple Choice

1. c   2. a   3. a

> **Note:**
>
> *There is no stated relationship between the diabetes mellitus and the iritis; therefore, the answer is a.*

4. c	10. c	16. c
5. b	11. a	17. c
6. b	12. a	18. c
7. a	13. c	19. a
8. b	14. a	20. d
9. d	15. b	

Coding Practice I: Diseases

286.0	21. Classical <u>hemophilia</u>
V53.31	22. <u>Fitting</u> of cardiac pacemaker
779.4	23. Gray <u>syndrome</u> from chloramphenicol administration in newborn
E985.1	24. Injury by shotgun, undetermined whether accidental or intentional (<u>shooting</u>)

> **Note:**
>
> *In the ICD-9-CM Index to External Causes and Injuries, go to main term* Shooting *and locate subterm* stated as undetermined whether accidental or intentional.

564.1	25. Irritable bowel <u>syndrome</u>
174.9	26. Malignant <u>neoplasm</u>, breast

> **Note:**
>
> *In the ICD-9-CM Index, go to the Neoplasm Table and locate the main term* Breast; *then locate code 174.9 in the Primary column.*

836.63	27. Medial <u>dislocation</u> of tibia, proximal end, open
E814.9	28. Motor vehicle traffic <u>accident</u> involving a collision with a pedestrian
300.14	29. <u>Multiple</u> personality
787.01	30. <u>Nausea</u> with vomiting
V14.0	31. Personal <u>history</u> of penicillin allergy
482.32	32. <u>Pneumonia</u> due to streptococcus, group B
714.31	33. Polyarticular juvenile rheumatoid <u>arthritis</u>, acute
753.14	34. <u>Polycystic</u> kidney, autosomal recessive
244.0	35. Postsurgical <u>hypothyroidism</u>
416.0	36. Pulmonary <u>arteriosclerosis</u>
134.1	37. Sand flea <u>infestation</u>
634.12	38. Spontaneous <u>abortion</u>, complicated by excessive hemorrhage, complete
651.31, V27.3	39. Twin <u>pregnancy</u> with loss of one fetus (delivered)
618.1	40. Uterine <u>prolapse</u>, first degree

Coding Practice II: Procedures

41.02	41. Allogenic bone marrow <u>transplant</u> with purging
01.14	42. <u>Biopsy</u>, brain (open)
77.52	43. <u>Bunionectomy</u> with soft tissue correction and arthrodesis
35.92	44. <u>Creation</u> of conduit between right ventricle and pulmonary artery
69.01	45. Dilation and curettage for <u>termination of pregnancy</u>
52.01	46. <u>Drainage</u> of pancreatic cyst by catheter
85.24	47. <u>Excision</u> of ectopic breast tissue
73.01	48. <u>Induction</u> of labor by artificial rupture of membranes
06.92	49. <u>Ligation</u> of thyroid vessels
57.12	50. <u>Lysis</u> of intraluminal adhesions with incision into bladder
22.31	51. Radical maxillary <u>antrotomy</u>
00.54	52. <u>Replacement</u> of cardiac resynchronization defibrillator pulse generator device only
19.6	53. Revision of <u>tympanoplasty</u>
11.42	54. <u>Therocauterization</u> of corneal lesion
60.96	55. Transurethral <u>destruction</u> of prostate tissue using microwave thermotherapy

Chapter 5
ICD-9-CM Hospital Inpatient Coding

HOSPITAL INPATIENT CODING ANSWER FORM

Copy and provide the form to students for their use in assigning codes to hospital inpatient case scenarios and records. Using the form will facilitate students' understanding of diagnosis and procedure sequencing.

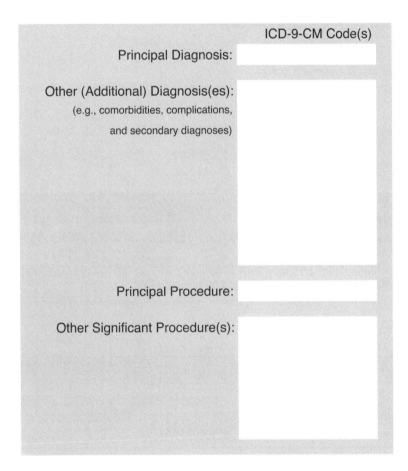

ICD-9-CM Code(s)

Principal Diagnosis:

Other (Additional) Diagnosis(es):
(e.g., comorbidities, complications, and secondary diagnoses)

Principal Procedure:

Other Significant Procedure(s):

EXERCISE 5.1 – ACUTE CARE FACILITIES (HOSPITALS)

1. acute care facility (ACF)
2. ancillary services
3. single hospitals; multihospital systems
4. bed size (or bed count)
5. short-term (or acute)
6. long-term (or long-term acute)
7. four

> **Note:**
>
> The month of May has 31 days. Count the day of admission, May 30, plus the remaining days through June 3 (May 31, June 1, and June 2). Do not count June 3 because it is the day of discharge.

8. nonacute

9. rehabilitation

10. hospitalists

11. intermediate care facility (ICF)

EXERCISE 5.2 – INPATIENT HOSPITAL CODING GUIDELINES – SEQUENCING INPATIENT DIAGNOSES AND PROCEDURES

Matching

1. b	5. g	9. e
2. h	6. i	10. c
3. f	7. d	
4. a	8. j	

Coding Diagnoses and Procedures

> **Note:**
>
> Procedure codes are not assigned for ancillary tests (e.g., laboratory tests and x-rays) in the case scenarios because such codes do not impact DRG assignment or the reimbursement amount for an inpatient case. However, because some hospitals do assign codes to ancillary tests (even though codes assigned do not impact the level of reimbursement received), students should be alerted to this practice.

11. 042,136.3,112.0,33.24

> **Note:**
>
> Chapter-specific coding guidelines provide instruction to sequence code 042 (AIDS) as the principal diagnosis, with AIDS-related conditions sequenced as other additional diagnoses. The bronchoscopy procedure was performed for the purpose of taking cell washings as a type of biopsy.

12. 433.11,784.5,342.91

> **Note:**
>
> The patient was admitted for treatment of the carotid artery occlusion with cerebral infarction (433.11), which is the principal diagnosis. When codes from categories 430–437 (e.g., 433.11) are assigned, additional codes are assigned to identify any sequelae present, such as dysphasia (784.5) and hemiparesis (342.91). Once the patient has completed initial treatment or is discharged from care, codes from category 438 are assigned to classify the late effects of cerebrovascular disease codes for dysphasia (438.12) and hemiparesis (438.21). The CT scan (87.03) does not impact the DRG reimbursement rate; therefore, that code is not assigned.

13. 813.42, E882, E849.0, 93.54

Note:

The ICD-9-CM Index to Diseases entry for "Fracture" includes subterm radius (alone) (closed) *and 2nd qualifier* lower end or extremity (distal end) (lower epiphysis), *which directs the coder to assign 813.42 (after verifying it in the Tabular List of Diseases). To locate the external cause of injury codes, go to main term* Fall, falling (accidental) *in the Index to External Causes of Injury and Poisonings and subterm* roof (through) *to locate code E882. Then go to main term* Accident (to), *subterm* occurring (at) (in) *and 2nd qualifier* home *to locate code E849.0. The splint application (93.54) code does not impact the DRG reimbursement rate; therefore, that code is not assigned.*

14. 250.61, 250.81, 357.2, 707.15, 785.4, 84.12

Note:

Chapter-specific coding guidelines provide instruction that the diabetes code is to be sequenced as the principal diagnosis for a condition such as "diabetic foot ulcers due to type 1 diabetic peripheral neuropathy" (250.61, 250.81). The manifestations of the diabetic peripheral neuropathy are reported as other additional diagnosis codes: 357.2 (peripheral neuropathy) and 707.15 (toe ulcer) and 785.4 (gangrene). To assign the procedure code, go to main term Amputation, forefoot *in the Index to Procedures and assign code 84.12 (after verifying the code in the Tabular List of Procedures).*

15. 345.41

Note:

To assign the principal diagnosis code, go to main term Epilepsy *in the Index to Diseases and locate subterm* partial (focalized), *2nd qualifier* with, *and 3rd qualifier* impairment of consciousness *to assign 345.41 (after verifying the code in the Tabular List of Diseases).*

REVIEW

Multiple Choice

1. a	8. b	15. c
2. b	9. b	16. b
3. a	10. b	17. c
4. b	11. d	18. c
5. a	12. c	19. a
6. c	13. a	20. d
7. b	14. d	

Coding Practice I: Hospital Inpatient Cases

> **Note:**
> - Coding rationales are included for each case to provide direction about assigning codes.
> - Procedure codes are not assigned for ancillary tests (e.g., laboratory tests and x-rays) in the case scenarios because such codes do not impact DRG assignment or the reimbursement amount for an inpatient case. However, because some hospitals do assign codes to ancillary tests (even though codes assigned do not impact the level of reimbursement received), students should be alerted about this practice.

21. 038.42, 995.91, 276.51, 402.91, 428.0

> **Note:**
> - The patient was admitted with symptoms of fever, myalgia, arthralgia, tachycardia, and dehydration. The physician suspected that the patient was septic and ordered a blood culture test, which was positive for Escherichia coli. Therefore, septicemia (038.42) is reported as the principal diagnosis. ICD-9-CM category code 038 contains an instructional note that states, "Use additional code for systemic inflammatory response syndrome (SIRS) 995.91-995-92." This means that code 995.91 is reported as an other (additional) diagnosis code.
> - Other diagnoses documented in the final diagnosis that are assigned codes include dehydration (276.51), hypertensive heart disease (402.91), and congestive heart failure (428.0). These diagnoses were treated with "routine medications" during the admission.
> - Do not assign a code to the "positive blood culture, Escherichia coli" diagnosis because it is included in the septicemia diagnosis.
> - Do not assign a code to the "pulmonary edema" diagnosis because that would be considered overcoding. The code reported for congestive heart failure (428.0) contains the following instruction: "INCLUDES: acute pulmonary edema with congestive heart failure."

22. 038.11, 995.92, 785.52, 584.9, 276.51, 691.0

> **Note:**
> - When septic shock is documented as a discharge diagnosis, report the code for septicemia (038.11) as the principal diagnosis. ICD-9-CM category code 038 contains an instructional note that states, "Use additional code for systemic inflammatory response syndrome (SIRS) 995.91-995-92." This means that code 995.91 is reported as an other (additional) diagnosis code.
> - This patient also was diagnosed as having septic shock, to which 785.52 is assigned as an other (additional) diagnosis code.
> - In addition, make sure you assign a code for any organ dysfunction; in this case, assign code 584.9 to acute renal failure.
> - Then assign a code for dehydration (276.51) and diaper rash (691.0).

23. 197.0, 157.0, 244.9, 250.00, 32.39

> **Note:**
>
> - When a patient is admitted for a primary malignant neoplasm with metastasis and treatment is directed toward the secondary site only, the secondary neoplasm code (197.0) is assigned as the principal diagnosis. The primary malignant neoplasm code (157.0) is assigned as an other (additional) diagnosis code.
> - In this case, codes for hypothyroidism (244.9) and diabetes (250.00) are also assigned.
> - Assign code 32.39 for the left lower lobe lung resection procedure.

24. 153.3, 197.0, 414.01, 412, 496

> **Note:**
>
> - Assign code 153.3 (carcinoma of sigmoid colon) as the principal diagnosis.
> - Assign code 197.0 (probable metastatic bronchogenic carcinoma) as an other (additional) diagnosis because a suspected carcinoma that receives inpatient treatment is coded as if confirmed. When a primary carcinoma metastasizes from its place of origin, the metastasized site is coded as a secondary neoplasm.
> - Chronic conditions that were medically managed during the hospitalization are assigned these codes: coronary artery disease (414.01) and chronic obstructive disease (496). Because documentation indicates that the patient has coronary artery disease with no history of coronary artery bypass surgery, assign code 414.01 to that diagnosis.
> - Code 412 is assigned to a healed or old myocardial infarction.

25. 250.70, 785.4, 041.7, 041.4, 84.11

> **Note:**
>
> - Diabetic gangrene is coded as 250.70, diabetes with peripheral circulatory disorders. Fifth digit 0 is assigned to indicate that the diabetes was not stated as uncontrolled.
> - An additional code is assigned to identify the manifestation; and in this case, the manifestation is gangrene (785.4).
> - Additional codes are also assigned to identify the bacterial agent in diseases classified elsewhere, so assign codes 041.7 (Pseudomonas) and 041.4 (Escherichia coli).
> - Assign code 84.11 for metatarsal amputation of the left great toe.

26. 244.9, 280.8, 532.30, 715.96

> **Note:**
>
> - Hypothyroidism is the condition established after study to be chiefly responsible for the patient's admission to the hospital. Thus, hypothyroidism (244.9) is reported as the principal diagnosis.
> - The iron deficiency anemia (280.8) is sequenced as an other (additional) diagnosis; it was due to hypothyroidism.
> - A code is assigned for the duodenal ulcer (532.30), and a code is assigned for osteoarthritis of the knee (715.96). Both the duodenal ulcer and osteoarthritis were treated during this admission.
> - The transfusion of packed red blood cells (99.04) does not impact the DRG reimbursement rate; therefore, that code is not assigned.

27. 282.62, 517.3

> **Note:**
> - Assign code 282.62 for sickle cell disease in crisis as the principal diagnosis.
> - Assign an other (additional) code for acute chest syndrome (517.3) to identify the type of crisis.

28. 285.22, 174.9, 198.5, 197.7, 244.9, V58.69, 99.04

> **Note:**
> - When an admission is for treatment of anemia due to a malignancy and only the anemia is treated, assign the code for anemia as the principal diagnosis. Anemia in neoplastic disease is coded as 285.22 and sequenced as principal diagnosis because it is the condition responsible for admission.
> - The underlying chronic conditions are coded as other (additional) diagnoses: carcinoma of breast (174.9) with metastases to bone and liver (197.7, 198.5) and hypothyroidism (244.9). These chronic conditions are underlying causes of the anemia. Code V58.69 is reported for long-term current use of other medications (e.g., chemotherapy).
> - The transfusion of packed red blood cells (99.04) does not impact the DRG reimbursement rate; however, that code may be reported.

29. 965.61, 427.1, 311, V62.0, V62.81, E950.0, E849.0

> **Note:**
> - If an overdose of a drug was intentionally taken, it is coded as a poisoning. Sequence the poisoning code first (965.61), followed by a code for the manifestation (427.1).
> - Codes V62.0 (unemployment) and V62.81 (relationship problems) provide additional information about the patient's status.
> - E codes are also assigned in this case to indicate that the poisoning was a suicide attempt (E950.5) and that the incident occurred at home (E849.0).
> - Assign a code for depression (311) as an other (additional) diagnosis.

30. 296.22, 94.27

> **Note:**
> - Involutional psychotic reaction is assigned 296.22 as the principal diagnosis. Fifth digit 2 is assigned because the physician stated that the reaction was moderate.
> - An other (additional) code for the depression is not assigned because it is implicit in the involutional psychotic reaction diagnosis.
> - The electroconvulsive therapy (94.27) does not impact the DRG reimbursement rate; however, that code may be reported.

31. 331.0, 294.11, 492.8, 250.00

> **Note:**
> - When coding Alzheimer's disease (331.0), assign an additional code for associated behavioral disturbances (294.10–294.11). "Dementia in conditions classified elsewhere" has been expanded to identify the presence or absence of behavioral disturbances. In this case, code 294.11 is assigned to identify that the patient was having behavioral disturbances (e.g., aggressive behavior and wandering). When assigning code 294.11, first code the underlying physical condition (331.0).
> - Then assign other (additional) codes for emphysema (492.8) and type 2 diabetes mellitus, controlled (250.00).

32. 435.9, 182.0, V58.69, 599.0, 041.3

> **Note:**
> - The patient was admitted with dizziness, weakness, and nystagmus, which are symptoms of the transient ischemic attack diagnosed by the physician. The transient ischemic attack (TIA) (435.9) is sequenced as the principal diagnosis. The symptoms are not coded because they are associated with the principal diagnosis of TIA.
> - The patient is currently being treated for the endometrial carcinoma; therefore, an other (additional) diagnosis is assigned for the carcinoma (182.0).
> - Report code V58.69 for long-term current administration of other medications (e.g., chemotherapy).
> - Assign a code for the urinary tract infection (599.0), with an additional code to identify the organism, Klebsiella pneumoniae (041.3).
> - The gait training physical therapy (93.22) code does not impact the DRG reimbursement rate; therefore, that code is not assigned.

33. 401.9, 444.81, 438.22, 438.11, 427.31

> **Note:**
> - Hypertension (401.9) is reported as the principal diagnosis. Assign hypertension to category 401 with the appropriate fourth digit to indicate malignant (.1), benign (.0), or unspecified (.9). Do not assign fourth digit .0 or .1 unless "malignant" or "benign" is documented in the patient record. (There is no documented cause-and-effect relationship between the hypertension and possible iliofemoral emboli; therefore, combination code 405.99 is *not* assigned.)
> - Assign possible iliofemoral emboli (444.81) as an other (additional) diagnosis. For inpatient hospitalizations, conditions stated as "possible" are coded as established diagnoses.
> - Codes from category 438 are assigned to indicate conditions classifiable to categories 430–437 as the cause of late effects. These include neurological deficits that persist after initial onset of the condition.
> - Assign an additional diagnosis code (427.31) for atrial fibrillation.

34. 410.11, 401.9, 272.0, 278.01

> **Note:**
>
> - Assign code 410.11 to acute anterior wall myocardial infarction as the principal diagnosis. Fifth digit 1 designates the first episode of care for a newly diagnosed myocardial infarction.
> - Additional diagnosis codes for chest pain and diaphoresis are not assigned because they are considered components of the myocardial infarction. Such symptoms integral to a myocardial infarction are not coded.
> - Assign 401.9 to hypertension as an other (additional) diagnosis. Assign hypertension to category 401 with the appropriate fourth digit to indicate malignant (.1), benign (.0), or unspecified (.9). Do not assign fourth digit .0 or .1 unless "malignant" or "benign" is documented in the patient record.
> - Other (additional) diagnosis codes are also assigned for hypercholesterolemia (272.0) and morbid obesity (278.01).

35. 466.0, 280.1, 787.01

> **Note:**
>
> - The patient was admitted due to symptoms of bronchitis and pneumonia. Pneumonia was ruled out. Therefore, assign code 466.0 to acute bronchitis as the principal diagnosis.
> - Do not code the cough because it is included in the diagnosis, bronchitis.
> - The meningitis also is not coded because it is no longer being medically managed.
> - Assign additional diagnosis codes for the nutritional anemia due to poor dietary iron intake (280.1) and nausea and vomiting (787.01) because they were treated during the hospitalization.

36. 491.22, 429.2, 411.1, 424.0

> **Note:**
>
> - The patient was admitted with shortness of breath and chest pain. The increasing chest pain was due to the chronic obstructive pulmonary disease with acute bronchitis; and when acute bronchitis is documented with chronic obstructive pulmonary disease, code 491.22 is assigned and sequenced as the principal diagnosis.
> - Do not assign an other (additional) diagnosis code for acute bronchitis (466.0). Do not assign a code for the respiratory distress because it is included in the code for the chronic obstructive pulmonary disease.
> - When the cause of the angina is clearly documented, sequence the cause before the appropriate angina code. In this case, progressive angina (411.1) is sequenced as an other (additional) code after the underlying cause of arteriosclerotic cardiovascular disease (429.2).
> - Also assign a code (424.0) for mitral insufficiency as an other (additional) diagnosis.

37. 153.3, 560.89, 332.0, 46.03, 96.07

> **Note:**
>
> - When a patient is admitted with a bowel obstruction due to sigmoid carcinoma, assign 153.3 as the principal diagnosis and sequence code 560.89, other intestinal obstruction, as an other (additional) diagnosis.
> - Do not assign a code for the abdominal distention because it is a symptom of the bowel obstruction.
> - Assign code 332.0 as an other (additional) diagnosis to Parkinson's disease.
> - Assign procedure codes to the loop colostomy (46.03) and insertion of the nasogastric tube (96.07). Sequence the loop colostomy as the principal procedure.

38. 532.30, 532.70, 553.3, 575.6, 733.00, 724.02

> **Note:**
>
> - If the same condition is described as both acute and chronic, code both the acute (532.30) and chronic (532.70) condition, sequencing the acute condition first. Assign fifth digit 0 for the acute and chronic ulcer to identify the ulcer as being without obstruction.
> - Do *not* assign a code for the abdominal pain because it is a symptom of the ulcer. Assign additional diagnosis codes for the hiatal hernia (553.3), gallbladder polyps (575.6), osteoporosis (733.00), and lumbar spinal stenosis (724.02).

39. 584.9, 276.51, 285.21, 585.6

> **Note:**
>
> - When a patient is diagnosed with acute renal failure and dehydration and the only treatment is intravenous hydration, it is appropriate to assign the code for acute renal failure (584.9) as the principal diagnosis. In most cases, intravenous hydration corrects the acute renal failure. The fact that the renal function was not investigated does not affect the code assignment.
> - Assign an other (additional) diagnosis code (276.51) for the dehydration.
> - Assign an other (additional) diagnosis code (285.21) for the anemia due to end-stage renal disease (585.6).
> - The transfusion of packed red blood cells code (99.04) does not impact the DRG reimbursement rate; therefore, that code is not assigned.

40. 600.90, 724.79, 401.9, 60.29

> **Note:**
>
> - Assign diagnosis code 600.90, benign prostatic hyperplasia, as the principal diagnosis. Fifth digit 0 is assigned to indicate the absence of urinary obstruction.
> - Assign an other (additional) diagnosis code for coccygodynia (724.79), which was evaluated and treated during the patient's stay.
> - Assign diagnosis code 401.9 for the hypertension that was under medical management.
> - Assign procedure code 60.29 for the transurethral resection of the prostate.

41. 620.2, 218.9, 617.9

> **Note:**
>
> - When two or more interrelated conditions meet the definition of principal diagnosis, either condition may be sequenced first as long as official coding guidelines do not indicate otherwise. Because it was determined that both the ovarian cyst (620.2) and the uterine fibroid (218.9) resulted in the patient's admission, either condition may be sequenced as the principal diagnosis.
> - Assign an other (additional) diagnosis code for the possible endometriosis (617.9). If a diagnosis at the time of hospital discharge is qualified as "possible," code the condition as if it were an established diagnosis.

42. 634.11, 69.02

Note:

- Diagnosis code 634.11 is assigned as the principal diagnosis for a spontaneous abortion with excessive bleeding. A fifth digit is required for abortion category 634. Fifth digit 1, incomplete, indicates that not all of the products of conception were expelled from the uterus.
- Procedure code 69.02 is assigned for dilatation and curettage following an abortion.

43. 660.11, 653.41, 661.21, V27.0, 74.1

Note:

- When a patient undergoes a cesarean delivery, the reason for the cesarean delivery is sequenced as the principal diagnosis. In this case, the cause is "obstructed labor." Two codes are reported for an obstructed labor. First code the obstructed labor (660.11), followed by the code for the cause of the obstruction. In this case, the cause is borderline cephalopelvic disproportion (653.41). To assist you in proper sequencing of the codes, category code 653 contains an instructional note that states, "Code first any obstructed labor" and category code 660.1 contains an instructional note that states, "Use additional code from 653.0-653.9." Fifth digit 1 is assigned to indicate "delivered, with or without mention of antepartum (before birth) condition."
- Diagnosis code 661.21, failure to progress, is assigned as an other (additional) diagnosis.
- A code from category V27, outcome of delivery, is always reported on maternal delivery records. It is always sequenced as an other (additional) diagnosis. In this case, V27.0 is coded to indicate that the outcome of delivery was a single liveborn.
- Assign procedure code 74.1 for the low cervical cesarean section.

44. 727.41, V25.2, 706.2, 82.21, 63.73, 21.32

Note:

- Assign diagnosis code 727.41, ganglion cyst of joint, as the principal diagnosis because it is the condition after study that occasioned the admission to the hospital.
- Assign code V25.2 for the other (additional) diagnosis of sterilization.
- Assign code 706.2 for the other (additional) diagnosis of cyst, skin of the nose.
- Assign procedure codes 82.21 (excision of ganglion cyst), 63.73 (bilateral vasectomy), and 21.32 (excision, lesion, skin of nose).

45. 707.07, 785.4, 041.11, 84.15

Note:

- Assign diagnosis code 707.07, decubitus ulcer of the heel, as the principal diagnosis.
- Code 785.4 (gangrene) is assigned as an additional diagnosis to identify the presence of gangrene and cellulitis. A separate cellulitis code is not assigned as it is inclusive in the code for the gangrene.
- Assign an additional diagnosis code to identify the Staphylococcus aureus infection (041.11).
- Assign procedure code 84.15, below-the-knee amputation, as the principal procedure.
- The whirlpool physical therapy treatment (93.32) code does not impact the DRG reimbursement rate; therefore, that code is not assigned.

46. 996.78, 458.29, 998.59, 041.4, E878.1, E878.8, 78.65, 93.24

Note:

- Diagnosis "painful Gouffon pins" is coded as a complication due to presence of other internal fixation device (996.78). Subcategory code 996.7 classifies the pain, and fifth digit 8 indicates that the pain is due to presence of the pin.
- Do *not* assign an other (additional) code for "pain" because that symptom is included in the 996.78 code.
- Assign E878.1 as an other (additional) diagnosis code to indicate that this complication was due to the surgical procedure, implant of an internal orthopedic device.
- Assign diagnosis code 458.29 as an other (additional) diagnosis code for postoperative hypotension.
- Assign code 998.59 as an other (additional) diagnosis code for the postoperative wound infection and assign code 041.4 for Escherichia coli as an other (additional) diagnosis to indicate the organism.
- Assign E878.8 as an other (additional) diagnosis to classify the complications due to surgical operation for the removal of the pin.
- Assign code 78.65 as the principal procedure code for removal of the pin.
- The gait training with a walker (93.24) code does not impact the DRG reimbursement amount; however, it may be reported.

47. 715.96, 81.54, 93.24

Note:

- Degenerative arthritis is coded to category 715.9, with fifth digit 6 assigned to indicate that the knee is the site of the arthritis (715.96).
- Do *not* assign a code to the knee pain because it is included in the arthritis diagnosis.
- Assign code 81.54 for total knee replacement as the principal procedure.
- The gait training with a walker (93.24) code does not impact the DRG reimbursement amount; however, it may be reported.

48. V30.00, 758.1, 764.09, 749.23, 755.01, 752.61, 756.3, 756.14, 753.3

Note:

- The appropriate code from the V30–V39 series is sequenced as the principal diagnosis. In this case, the principal diagnosis code is V30.00 for single liveborn, baby born in the hospital, and no cesarean section.
- When congenital condition(s) are diagnosed during the hospital episode in which an infant is born, appropriate code(s) from Chapter 14 of the ICD-9-CM coding manual are assigned as other (additional) diagnoses. The following codes are assigned as other (additional) diagnoses:
  - Trisomy 13(758.1)
  - Small for dates (764.09)
  - Cleft lip and palate, complete (749.23)
  - Polydactyly of the fingers (755.01)
  - Hypospadias (752.61)
  - Extra rib (756.3)
  - Hemivertebra (756.14)
  - Dextroversion, left kidney (753.3)

49. 745.0, 780.2

Note:

- Congenital aortic septal defect is assigned code 745.0 and sequenced as the principal diagnosis.
- Code 780.2 is assigned to syncope as an other (additional) diagnosis.
- Do not assign codes for the shortness of breath, fatigue, and vague chest pain because they are symptoms of (and included in) the principal diagnosis code.

50. V30.00, 765.17, 765.26, 779.5

Note:

- When coding the birth of an infant, assign a code from category V30–V39 as the principal diagnosis. In this case, assign V30.00 for single liveborn, born in the hospital, no cesarean section.
- The diagnosis of "premature infant" is coded to subcategory 765.1, with a fifth digit to indicate the infant's birth weight in grams. In this case, assign 765.17 because the infant weighed 1760 grams.
- Subcategory 765.1 includes a note to "use an additional code for the weeks of gestation." This means that an other (additional) diagnosis code is assigned from subcategory 765.2, with the appropriate fifth-digit code to indicate the weeks of gestation. In this case, assign 765.26 to indicate 32 weeks' gestation.
- Assign an other (additional) diagnosis code for withdrawal symptoms (779.5).

51. V30.01, 774.6, 99.83

Note:

- When coding the birth of an infant, assign a code from categories V30–V39 as the principal diagnosis. For this case, assign code V30.01, single liveborn, born in the hospital, cesarean section delivery.
- Assign code 774.6 to hyperbilirubinemia as an other (additional) diagnosis.
- The phototherapy treatment of a newborn (99.83) code does not impact the DRG reimbursement amount; however, it may be reported.

52. 780.31, 381.01

Note:

- Assign code 780.31 to febrile seizure as the principal diagnosis because it is the condition that occasioned the admission to the hospital.
- Do *not* assign a code to the fever because it is included in the febrile seizure code.
- Assign code 381.01 for the acute serous otitis media as an other (additional) diagnosis.

53. 789.03

Note:

The patient was admitted to the hospital due to her abdominal pain, and a definitive diagnosis was never made for the cause of the abdominal pain. Therefore, assign code 789.03 as the principal diagnosis for right lower quadrant abdominal pain. The fifth digit 3 is assigned to identify that the pain was in the right lower quadrant.

54. 943.21, 942.25, 945.26, 948.00, E924.0, E849.0

> **Note:**
>
> - The principal diagnosis code reflects the highest degree of burn when a patient is admitted with more than one burn. Because the patient's burns were all second-degree, sequence either 943.21 (second-degree burn of the forearm), 942.25 (second-degree burn of the vulva), or 945.26 (second-degree burn of the thigh) as the principal diagnosis.
> - Then assign a code from category 948 to classify "burns according to extent of body surface involved." Category 948 codes are assigned when it is necessary to provide data for evaluating burn mortality. Assign diagnosis code 948.00 to indicate the patient had burns over 7 percent of her body.
> - Assign E924.0 to indicate that the burn was due to a hot liquid and E849.0 to indicate that the accident occurred at home.
> - The nonexcisional debridement of burns (86.28) does not impact the DRG reimbursement amount; therefore, that code is not assigned.
> - Do *not* assign a code for the placement of dressings.

55. 823.32, 813.42, 873.64, E812.2, 79.36, 25.51

> **Note:**
>
> - Codes for multiple fractures are sequenced according to severity, and the code for an open fracture is sequenced before a closed fracture. For this case, sequence diagnosis code 823.32, open fracture of the tibia with fibula, as the principal diagnosis.
> - Assign an other (additional) diagnosis code for closed fracture of the distal radius (813.42).
> - Assign an other (additional) diagnosis code for tongue laceration (873.64). The laceration of the tongue is coded "without mention of complication" because there was no mention of delayed healing, delayed treatment, foreign body, or infection.
> - Code E812.2 is assigned to indicate that the patient was the driver of a motorcycle that collided with a parked vehicle.
> - Assign procedure code 79.36 (open reduction, internal fixation of tibia/fibula) as the principal procedure.
> - Assign code 25.51 for the suture repair of the tongue laceration.
> - The casting (93.53) code does not impact the DRG reimbursement rate; therefore, that code is not assigned.

Chapter 6
ICD-9-CM Outpatient and Physician Office Coding

EXERCISE 6.1 – OUTPATIENT CARE

1. outpatient (or ambulatory)
2. primary
3. primary care provider
4. ambulatory patients (or outpatients)
5. ambulatory surgery patients
6. emergency department patients (or emergency care patients)
7. observation patients
8. clinic
9. referred
10. triage

EXERCISE 6.2 – DIAGNOSTIC CODING AND REPORTING GUIDELINES FOR OUTPATIENT SERVICES – HOSPITAL-BASED AND PHYSICIAN OFFICE

1. skin lesion
2. shortness of breath
3. fractured humerus
4. gastroenteritis
5. urinary frequency
6. acute bronchitis
7. back pain
8. diabetes mellitus
9. outpatient chemotherapy
10. acute cholecystitis with cholelithiasis

EXERCISE 6.3 – ICD-9-CM CODING GUIDELINES FOR OUTPATIENT DIAGNOSTIC TESTS

1. intra-abdominal abscess
2. pulmonary nodule
3. wheezing
4. degenerative joint disease at L1 and L2
5. pneumonia due to Streptococcus, Group B

REVIEW

Multiple Choice

1. d	8. d	15. d
2. a	9. c	16. c
3. c	10. c	17. c
4. d	11. c	18. d
5. a	12. b	19. a
6. a	13. a	20. b
7. c	14. c	

Coding Practice

> **Note:**
> - Coding rationales are included for each case to provide direction about assigning codes.
> - ICD-9-CM codes are not assigned to procedures or services because HCPCS level II and CPT codes are assigned to outpatient procedures and services. (ICD-9-CM procedure codes are assigned to inpatient cases, as discussed in Chapter 5.)

Ambulatory Surgery Center (ASC)

21. 244.9

> **Note:**
> Do not assign a code for asthma because that condition was not medically managed during this outpatient encounter. Providers medically manage conditions when they evaluate the condition, prescribe medications, order tests, and so on.

22. 211.1, V18.51

> **Note:**
> Assign code 211.1 even though the diagnosis documents "multiple" gastric polyps. Code V18.51 is assigned to classify the "past family history of polyposis."

23. V25.2

> **Note:**
> Do not assign a code for the chest pain or endocardial ischemia because these conditions were not medically managed during this outpatient encounter.

24. 550.90   25. V25.2, V61.5

Note:

This case scenario documents the patient complaint of multiparity. Thus, V61.5 is assigned as a secondary diagnosis code.

Chiropractic Office

26. 722.71   27. 847.0

Note:

Do not assign codes for the neck pain and stiffness because those are symptoms of the definitive diagnosis, acute cervical sprain.

28. 847.0, 724.5, 724.8

Note:

The numbness and tingling in her left arm is due to the cervical neck strain; therefore, do not assign codes for these symptoms. Code 724.5 is assigned for documented soreness of the upper back. The Index to Diseases instructs you to assign 724.8 for stiffness of the upper back. Note that this condition is not listed in the Tabular List of Diseases code description for 724.8; thus, this is an example of the trust-the-index coding convention.

29. 721.0

Note:

To assign code 721.0, refer to main term Osteoarthritis and subterm Spine, Spinal NEC (see also Spondylosis) 721.90. Next, refer to main term Spondylosis and subterm cervical, cervicodorsal 721.0. Verify code 721.0 in the tabular list.

30. 847.0, 724.5, 719.41, 784.0

Note:

Do not assign 719.49 (Pain in joint, multiple sites) for "shoulder and back pain" because it is classified in a different category than shoulder pain. If the patient had shoulder and elbow pain, assigning code 719.49 would be correct.

Hospital Emergency Department

31. 784.0   32. 719.41, E927, E849.9

Note:

The shoulder is a joint. Therefore, in the Index to Diseases, go to main term Pain, *subterm* joint, *and 2nd qualifier* shoulder *to assign the code (719.41).*

33. 490, 481

Note:

- Because the chest x-ray documents "slight increased density at right lower lobe," assign the code for "pneumonia, lobar." The radiologist who documents the x-ray report findings is a physician; so even though the attending physician did not document "lobar pneumonia" in the diagnosis statement, the x-ray report supports the code assignment for "lobar pneumonia."
- There is no documentation of the infectious organism; therefore, do not assign a code for the type of infection. (If performed, sputum culture results would document the infectious organism.)

34. 845.00   35. 883.0, E928.8, E849.9

Note:

Go to main term Wound *and subterm* finger *in the Index to Diseases to assign the code (883.0). There is no mention of a complication (e.g., infection of the puncture wound).*

Hospital Outpatient Department

36. V81.2, V17.49

Note:

- The patient's EKG was negative, which means she was not diagnosed as having cardiovascular disease. The nonspecific T-wave changes were explained as probably due to anxiety and positional changes during the procedure. Therefore, go to main term *Screening* and subterm *cardiovascular disease* in the Index to Diseases to assign the code (V81.2).
- Assign code V17.49 for "family history of cardiovascular disease."
- Do not assign code V71.7 because the patient did not present with cardiovascular symptoms. This patient underwent a screening EKG because of a family history of cardiovascular disease.

37. 710.0   38. 414.01

> **Note:**
>
> - There is no past history of coronary artery bypass graft surgery; therefore, assign the ASHD code (414.01) that describes "native coronary artery" as the type of vessel.
> - If documentation had been unclear as to whether the patient had a past history of CABG surgery, the ASHD subclassification code that describes "unspecified type of vessel, native or graft" would have been assigned.
> - If the patient had a past history of CABG surgery and documentation indicated that blockages were associated with previously grafted vessels, the ASHD subclassification code that describes "bypass graft" as the type of vessel would have been assigned.
> - If the patient had a past history of being the recipient of a transplanted heart and documentation indicated that blockages were associated with vessels of the transplanted heart, the ASHD subclassification code that describes "native vessel of the transplanted heart" as the type of vessel would have been assigned.

39. 428.0, V65.3, V65.42

> **Note:**
>
> *Codes V65.3 and V65.42 are assigned to classify "dietary surveillance and counseling" and "counseling on substance use and abuse," respectively.*

40. V56.0, 996.81, 753.0, E878.0

> **Note:**
>
> *The reason for this encounter is hemodialysis (V56.0), which is necessary because the patient's transplanted kidney failed (996.81). She was also born with just one kidney (753.0). Code E878.0 is assigned to classify the complication of the failed transplanted kidney.*

Hospital Same-Day Surgery

41. 474.0

> **Note:**
>
> *The first sentence of this case documents recurrent (or chronic) bouts of tonsillitis, and the diagnosis documents "diseased . . . adenoids." Thus, code 474.0 is reported.*

42. 600.00, 585.9, 599.0, 041.04

> **Note:**
>
> - There is no mention of urinary retention in the case scenario; therefore, assign code 600.00 for "benign prostatic hypertrophy."
> - Assign code 585.9 to "chronic renal insufficiency" because it was caused by the "benign prostatic hypertrophy."
> - Assign code 599.0 for "urinary tract infection" and make sure you assign a code (041.04) to identify the infectious organism (enterococcus).
> - "Anemia" and "pre-pyloric gastric ulcer" were not medically managed during this encounter; therefore, do not assign codes to these conditions.

43. 565.0, 455.6

> **Note:**
>
> - The patient underwent fissurectomy and hemorrhoidectomy, so assign codes for "anal fissure" (565.0) and "hemorrhoids" (455.6).
> - Although "obesity" is likely a contributing factor to the development of the anal fissure and hemorrhoids, there is no documentation that this condition was medically managed. Therefore, do not assign a code for obesity.

44. 241.9, 226

> **Note:**
>
> - There is no documentation of the type of "nodular colloid goiter," which means the unspecified code (241.9) is assigned.
> - "Degenerating follicular adenoma, right lobe of thyroid" is a benign neoplasm (226).

45. 634.91

> **Note:**
>
> An "incomplete abortion" is a miscarriage. The main term Miscarriage in the Index to Diseases contains the instruction to "see Abortion, spontaneous." When verifying subcategory code 634.9 in the Tabular List of Diseases, fifth digit 1 for "incomplete" is assigned.

Physician Office

46. 871.4

> **Note:**
>
> Main term Laceration and subterm cornea contains an instruction to "see Laceration, eyeball," which results in code 871.4.

47. 891.0

> **Note:**
>
> Go to main term Wound *and subterm* knee *in the Index to Diseases to assign the code (891.0). (There is no documentation of a complication, such as a wound infection.)*

48. 603.9   49. 883.0

> **Note:**
>
> The main term Laceration *in the Index to Diseases contains the instruction to "see also* Wound, open, by site." *Go to main term* Wound *and subterm* thumb *to assign the code (883.0). The word* nail *is a nonessential modifier enclosed in parentheses next to subterm* thumb *in the Index to Diseases. Therefore, assign 883.0 as a combination coded to the condition, "laceration, thumbnail and thumb, left."*

50. 729.81, 729.5

> **Note:**
>
> - The main term *Swollen* in the Index to Diseases contains the instruction to *"see also Swelling."* Therefore, go to main term *Swelling* and subterm *hand* in the Index to Diseases to assign the code (729.81).
> - Go to main term *Pain* and subterm *hand* in the Index to Diseases to assign code 729.5 for "hand . . . painful to touch."

Stand-Alone Radiology Center

51. 585.9, 996.74

> **Note:**
>
> - An "occluded dialysis access graft" is a complication of the access graft, which needs surgical repair (to clear the occlusion). Go to main term *Complication*, subterm *blood vessel graft,* and 2nd qualifier occlusion in the Index to Diseases to assign the code (996.74).
> - An occluded graft is *not* a mechanical complication of the blood vessel graft, which would be assigned a different code to describe the mechanical complication (e.g., torn graft or twisting of graft).

52. 575.8   53. 577.1

> **Note:**
>
> Do not assign an ICD-9-CM code to "stomach pain" because that is a symptom of the recurrent pancreatitis.

54. 788.30   55. 719.06, 836.0

> **Note:**
>
> • Go to main term *Effusion*, subterm *joint*, and 2nd qualifier *knee to* assign code 719.06.
> • Go to main term *Tear*, subterm *meniscus*, 2nd qualifier *medial*, and 3rd qualifier *posterior horn* in the Index to Diseases to assign the code (836.0) for "ruptures of posterior segment of right medial meniscus."

Stand-Alone Urgent Care Center

56. 913.0, 916.0, 881.01, 844.9, 845.00

> **Note:**
>
> • Main term *Abrasion* in the Index to Diseases contains an instruction to "see also *Injury, superficial, by site.*" Therefore, go to main term *Injury*, subterm *superficial*, and 2nd qualifier *arm* to assign code 913.0 (after selecting the fourth digit 0 from the Tabular List of Diseases).
> • Return to main term *Injury*, and subterm *superficial*; locate 2nd qualifier leg to assign code 916.0 (after selecting the fourth digit 0 from the Tabular List of Diseases).
> • Main term *Laceration* contains an instruction to "see also *Wound, open, by site.*" Therefore, go to main term *Wound* and subterm *elbow to* assign the code (881.01).
> • The condition "sprain, right knee, lower leg" is assigned combination code 844.9 (for knee and leg). A separate code (845.00) is assigned for "sprain, ankle."

57. 682.4,796.2

> **Note:**
>
> Code 796.2 is assigned to "elevated blood pressure reading" because the provider discussed the sign with the patient and made plans for follow-up treatment.

58. 720.2

> **Note:**
>
> Go to main term Inflammation, *subterm* joint, *and 2nd qualifier* sacroiliac to *assign the code (720.2).*

59. 706.2

> **Note:**
>
> Go to main term Cyst and subterm sebaceous to assign the code (706.2). There is no 2nd qualifier for "infected" or "right cheek."

60. 784.7

Chapter 7
HCPCS Level II National Coding System

EXERCISE 7.1 – OVERVIEW OF HCPCS

1. national
2. durable medical equipment, prosthetics, orthotics, supplies (DMEPOS)
3. level I
4. five
5. A–V

EXERCISE 7.2 – HCPCS LEVEL II CODES

1. HCPCS National Panel
2. Medicare Carriers Manual (MCM)
3. Medicare National Coverage Determinations Manual
4. HCPCS National Panel
5. American Dental Association (ADA)
6. DMEPOS dealer
7. outpatient PPS
8. annual
9. E1
10. modifiers

EXERCISE 7.3 – ASSIGNING HCPCS LEVEL II CODES

1. injection, medication
2. twice
3. once
4. supplies
5. Medicare
6. medications
7. table of contents
8. alphabetical first character
9. commercial payers
10. CPT

EXERCISE 7.4 - DETERMINING PAYER RESPONSIBILITY

1. c   5. c   9. c
2. b   6. b   10. c
3. a   7. b
4. b   8. a

REVIEW

Multiple Choice

1. c   8. d   15. c
2. d   9. a   16. c
3. b   10. d   17. a
4. .a   11. d   18. b
5. a   12. c   19. d
6. d   13. a   20. c
7. c   14. c

Coding Practice I

Transportation Services Including Ambulance (A0000–A0999)

> **Note:**
>
> The main term Ambulance *requires review of codes A0021–A0999 to locate the appropriate five-character HCPCS level II code and two-character modifier.*

21. A0433-PH

22. A0225-HH

23. A0429-RH

24. A0422-NH

25. A0130-EP

Medical and Surgical Supplies (A4000–A8999)

26. A4208-AG

27. A4246-TD

28. A4261

> **Note:**
>
> According to Encoder Pro Expert, code A4261 is exempt from adding a modifier to identify the type of practitioner who performed the procedure.

29. A4282-NU

30. A6410

Administrative, Miscellaneous and Investigational (A9000–A9999)

31. A9526

32. A9300-RR

33. A9528 × 2

34. A9700

35. A9153

Enteral and Parenteral Therapy (B4000–B9999)

36. B4224, B4224

37. B4155

38. B9002-NU

39. B4036-NU

40. B4224 × 2

Outpatient PPS (C1000–C9999)

41. C1717-AF

42. C1764-SC

43. C1789

44. C8905-LT

45. C1752-RT

Dental Procedures (D0000–D9999)

46. D3410

47. D1120

48. D5912

49. D2722

50. D7510

Durable Medical Equipment (E0100–E9999)

51. E0910

52. E0455

53. E0202

54. E0570

55. E0135-NU

Procedures/Professional Services (Temporary) (G0000–G9999)

56. G0307

57. Code deleted effective 12/31/08

58. G9016, G9016 × 2

59. G0104

60. G0252

Alcohol and/or Drug Abuse Treatment Services (H0001-H2037)

61. H0004-HJ × 2

62. H0035

63. H2013

64. H0045 × 3

65. H2032-GP × 2

Drugs Administered Other Than Oral Method (J0000–J9999)

66. J0706
67. J1550
68. J2501
69. J3265
70. J9000

Temporary Codes (K0000–K9999)

71. K0072-RP × 2
72. K0105
73. K0038 × 2
74. K0012-RR
75. K0603

Orthotic Procedures (L0000–L4999)

76. L0160
77. L0220
78. L0830
79. L3310 × 2
80. L1960-AV

Prosthetic Procedures (L5000–L9999)

81. L5150
82. L7025
83. L5000
84. L6825, L6895
85. L8030

Medical Services (M0000–M0301)

> **Note:**
>
> *Most HCPCS level II medical services codes are not typically reimbursed by third-party payers. These statements are provided for coding practice.*

86. M0064
87. M0075
88. M0300
89. M0301
90. M0076

Pathology and Laboratory Services (P0000–P9999)

91. P9612
92. P3000
93. P9045
94. P9019 × 2
95. P9010 × 2

Q Codes: Temporary Codes (Q0000–Q9999)

96. Q0083
97. Q3031
98. Q2017
99. Q4023
100. Q0112

Diagnostic Radiology Services (R0000–R5999)

Note:

HCPCS level II diagnostic radiology services codes are reported in addition to CPT radiology codes.

101. R0075-US
102. R0076-UR
103. R0075-UN

Temporary National Codes (Non-Medicare) (S0000–S9999)

104. S2142
105. S2202
106. S3708
107. S0400
108. S2055

National T Codes Established for State Medicaid Agencies (T1000–T9999)

109. T1027
110. T2101
111. T1502-TE
112. T1000-TD $\times$ 2
113. T2035

Vision Services (V0000–V2999)

114. V2208 $\times$ 2
115. V2025
116. V2744 $\times$ 2
117. V2785
118. V2626

Hearing Services (V5000–V5999)

119. V5010
120. V5140
121. V5245
122. V5240
123. V5268

Coding Practice II

124. J0456   Zithromax (azythromycin) 500 mg injection
     R0070   Chest x-ray by mobile service; one patient seen

> **Note:**
>
> Code R0070 is reported by the mobile x-ray service.

125. J1670   Injection, tetanus immune globulin, human, up to 250 mg
     E0112   Wooden crutches

> **Note:**
>
> Do not assign HCPCS level II code to the pHisoHex solution, sterile gauze, or paper tape. Those supplies are included in the provision of the evaluation and management service, which would be assigned a separate CPT code for this case.
>
> Do not assign HCPCS code J2001 for Xylocaine. Although lidocaine HCL is the generic name for Xylocaine, code J2001 is assigned when lidocaine HCL is injected for intravenous infusion.

Chapter 8
Introduction to CPT Coding

EXERCISE 8.1 – HISTORY OF CPT

1. b   3. a   5. c
2. e   4. d

EXERCISE 8.2 – OVERVIEW OF CPT

1. clinical providers   3. medical necessity   5. III
2. third-party payer   4. II

EXERCISE 8.3 – ORGANIZATION OF CPT

1. six
2. these codes are reported by all specialties
3. Anesthesia
4. vesiculotomy; complicated
5. Code 47560 is assigned for a surgical laparoscopy with guided transhepatic cholangiography, without biopsy. Code 47562 is assigned for a laparoscopic cholecystectomy.

EXERCISE 8.4 – CPT INDEX

1. T   3. F   5. F
2. F   4. T

EXERCISE 8.5 – CPT APPENDICES

1. d   6. b   11. k
2. a   7. b   12. e
3. f   8. h   13. i
4. l   9. j   14. m
5. g   10. c

EXERCISE 8.6 – CPT SYMBOLS

1. a   3. e   5. c
2. d   4. f   6. b

EXERCISE 8.7 – CPT SECTIONS, SUBSECTIONS, CATEGORIES, AND SUBCATEGORIES

1. F   3. T   5. F
2. F   4. T

EXERCISE 8.8 – CPT MODIFIERS

1. -80	5. -56	9. -50
2. -79	6. -55	10. -32
3. -25	7. -76	
4. -57	8. -51	

EXERCISE 8.9 – NATIONAL CORRECT CODING INITIATIVE

1. Medicare Part B claims
2. Outpatient Code Editor (OCE)
3. comprehensive/component; mutually exclusive
4. Advanced Beneficiary Notice (ABN); Notice of Exclusions from Medicare Benefits (NEMB)
5. unbundling

REVIEW

Multiple Choice

1. d	8. d	15. b
2. c	9. d	16. b
3. a	10. b	17. a
4. b	11. b	18. a
5. c	12. c	19. d
6. b	13. d	20. b
7. c	14. d	

Coding Practice

CPT Index

21.	Main term	Debridement
	Subterm	Skin
	2nd qualifier	Subcutaneous tissue
	3rd qualifier	Infected
	Code range	11004–11006
22.	Main term	Arthrodesis
	Subterm	Elbow
	Code range	24800–24802
		- or -
	Main term	Elbow
	Subterm	Arthrodesis
	Code range	24800–24802
23.	Main term	Kocher pylorectomy
	Cross-reference	See Gastrectomy; partial
	Main term	Gastrectomy
	Subterm	Partial
	Code range	43631–43635, 43845

24. Main term   Hysterectomy
    Subterm   Abdominal
    2nd qualifier   Resection of Ovarian Malignancy
    Code range   58951,58953–58956

25. Main term   PET
    Cross-reference   See Positron Emission Tomography
    Main term   Positron Emission Tomography (PET)
    Subterm   Brain
    Code range   78608–78609

CPT Appendices

26. 1007F— Assessment for use of anti-inflammatory or analgesic OTC (over-the-counter) medications.

27. Category   Dysmorphology
    Modifier   9N

28. three

> **Note:**
>
> *The patient underwent two nerve conduction studies, and the maximum number allowed is three. This means that the patient can return for an additional nerve conduction study.*

29. The gastroduodenal and proper hepatic arteries are third-order branches that branch from the celiac trunk, a first-order artery.

30. Code 43228 is included in the list of CPT codes that includes moderate (conscious) sedation, which means that a code from range 99143–99145 is *not* reported.

CPT Symbols

31. The flash (✗) symbol precedes code 90736, which means it is pending FDA approval.

32. The plus (✚) symbol precedes code 59525, which means it is an add-on code and modifier -51 is not added to the code.

33. The bull's-eye (◉) symbol precedes code 45380, which means that conscious sedation is included. Conscious sedation is not coded and reported separately.

34. The forbidden (⊘) symbol precedes code 31500, which means that modifier -51 is not added to the code.

35. The semicolon (;) symbol is included in the description of code 21480 to save space in CPT. The description of code 21480 is "closed treatment of temporomandibular dislocation; initial or subsequent." The description of code 21485 is "closed treatment of temporomandibular dislocation; complicated (e.g., recurrent requiring intermaxillary fixation or splinting), initial or subsequent. Thus, code 21480 must be referred back to as the common portion of the code description.

CPT Modifiers

36. Modifier -51 is added to code 12002 to indicate that multiple procedures were performed during the same operative session on the same day of service.

37. Modifier -50 is added to 30905 to indicate that a bilateral procedure was performed during the same operative session on the same day of service.

38. Modifier -26 (Professional Component) is added to the CPT code for the MRI.

39. Modifier -76 (Repeat Procedure by Same Physician) is added to code 56420.

40. Modifier -77 should be assigned to report a repeat procedure by another physician.

Chapter 9
CPT Evaluation and Management

EXERCISE 9.1 – OVERVIEW OF EVALUATION AND MANAGEMENT SECTION

1. Preventive Medicine Services
2. Emergency Department Services
3. history and examination
4. 5
5. place of service (POS)
6. type of service (TOS)
7. consultation
8. office
9. Consultations
10. Office or Other Outpatient Consultations

EXERCISE 9.2 – EVALUATION AND MANAGEMENT SECTION GUIDELINES

1. established
2. new
3. established
4. fractured pelvis
5. numbness, left foot

EXERCISE 9.3 – LEVELS OF EVALUATION AND MANAGEMENT SERVICES

1. a. 99204
   b. 99211
   c. 99222
   d. 99245
   e. 99283
2. a. yes
   b. 99284-25
3. a. no
   b. no code
4. extent of history, extent of examination, and complexity of medical decision making
5. three
6. two out of three

7. counseling, coordination of care, nature of presenting problem, and time
8. a. Office or Other Outpatient Services, Established Patient
   b. 99213
9. To assign the E/M code, the following is determined:
   a. established (The patient was seen in the office for "routine three-month follow-up.")
   b. expanded problem focused

> **Note:**
>
> Chief complaint is "follow-up for evaluation and management type 2 diabetes mellitus and hypertension." According to the 1997 E/M documentation guidelines, two elements of the history of present illness (HPI) were documented: quality (stable) and severity (home monitoring), which means that a brief HPI was performed. Documentation of the review of system (ROS) included five body areas/systems (chest pain—cardiovascular; headache—neurologic; extremities—musculoskeletal; shortness of breath—respiratory; and visual changes—eyes), making this an extended ROS. Since there is no documentation of past, family, or social history, the highest extent of history that can be selected is expanded problem focused.

   c. expanded problem focused

> **Note:**
>
> According to the 1997 E/M documentation guidelines, elements are counted as follows: constitutional (1) (blood pressure, weight, and pulse count as one element); eyes (1) (pupils equal, round, and reactive to light and accommodation); ears, nose, and throat (2) (external auditory canals/tympanic membranes negative; oropharynx benign); neck (2) (supple; no bruits, jugular venous distention, or thyromegaly) (maximum of two elements can be identified for neck); respiratory (2) (breath sounds clear to auscultation and percussion; auscultation, or listening to the lungs, revealed no rubs, rales, rhonchi, or wheezing) (maximum of four elements can be identified for respiratory); cardiovascular (3) (no click, gallop, irregularity, murmur, or rub; distal pulses intact; no edema); musculoskeletal (1) (no cyanosis, clubbing); and neurological (2) (deep tendon reflexes within normal limits and symmetrical; no decreased lower extremity sensation noted). A total of 14 elements were documented, which means that an expanded problem-focused examination was performed. (Although more than 12 elements were documented, the physician did not perform a comprehensive examination, which would have required examination of all elements in at least 9 body areas/organs.)

   d. moderate complexity

> **Note:**
>
> The number of diagnoses and management options documented is multiple because two diagnoses and management options must be considered. The amount and complexity of data to be reviewed are minimal because just lab tests are considered. The risk of complications and/or morbidity or mortality is moderate because of the documented prescription drug therapy for two stable chronic illnesses. Since the complexity of medical decision making is determined by the two highest of the three options, the level for this encounter is moderate complexity.

e. The E/M code is 99213.

> **Note:**
>
> *An expanded problem-focused history, a detailed examination, and moderate complexity of medical decision making were documented. Because two of three key components determine the E/M level for an established patient visit, assign 99213. Code selection is based on extent of examination and complexity of medical decision making. (No contributory components, such as counseling or coordination of care, were documented.)*

10. 99254

EXERCISE 9.4 – EVALUATION AND MANAGEMENT CATEGORIES AND SUBCATEGORIES

1. F	11. T	21. F
2. F	12. T	22. T
3. T	13. F	23. F
4. F	14. T	24. T
5. T	15. F	25. T
6. F	16. T	26. T
7. F	17. F	27. F
8. T	18. T	28. F
9. T	19. F	29. F
10. F	20. T	30. T

REVIEW

Multiple Choice

1. a	7. a	13. d
2. b	8. b	14. c
3. a	9. b	15. c
4. c	10. c	16. a
5. c	11. c	
6. b	12. d	

> **Note:**
>
> *The nursing facility patient is "recovering," which means that code 99307 is reported.*

17. a

18. b

19. a

20. b

Coding Practice

Office or Other Outpatient Services

21. 99213

> **Note:**
>
> An established patient requires two out of three key components be met or exceeded for a particular level of E/M service to be assigned. In this case, a problem-focused history was performed. (It is part of code 99212.) The examination and medical decision making are level 3 (code 99213). Since just two key components need to be met, the level 3 E/M code is assigned.

22. 99202

> **Note:**
>
> For a new patient, three out of three key components must be met or exceeded to assign an E/M code. Code 99202 requires an expanded problem-focused history and examination and straightforward medical decision making.

Hospital Observation Services

23. 99219

> **Note:**
>
> For initial hospital observation care, three out of three key components must be met or exceeded for a level to be assigned. In this case, documentation warrants assignment of a level 2 initial observation code.

24. 99218 (5/7), 99217 (5/8)

> **Note:**
>
> Two codes are assigned to this case: one for initial observation care and one for observation care discharge. For the initial observation care, three out of three key components must be met or exceeded to assign a level. For the discharge care, the physician must document a final exam, patient instructions, and discussion of the hospital stay.

Hospital Inpatient Services

25. 99222 (10/10), 99232 (10/11), 99232 (10/12), 99238 (10/13)

> **Note:**
>
> Four codes are required for this case. 99222 is the E/M code for initial hospital care level 2, 99232 reflects subsequent hospital care level 2, and 99238 reflects discharge day management 30 minutes or less.

26. 99233

> **Note:**
>
> *For an established patient, two out of three key components are required. For this case, the coder can use the detailed physical examination and the MDM of a high level. The detailed history does not have to be used to assign a subsequent hospital care E/M code.*

Consultations

27. 99242

> **Note:**
>
> *For office consultations with new patients, three out of three key components must be met or exceeded for a level to be assigned. For 99242, an expanded problem-focused history, expanded problem-focused exam, and medical decision making of a straightforward nature are the requirements.*

28. 99255

> **Note:**
>
> *Initial inpatient consultation codes require three out of three key components be met in order to assign a specific level. A comprehensive history, comprehensive exam, and MDM of high level would code to 99255.*

Emergency Department Services

29. 99285

> **Note:**
>
> *The presenting problem in this patient warrants a high E/M level. The diagnoses of shortness of breath and chest pain are critical medical issues. Since no time was documented by the physician, critical care service code 99291 or 99292 could not be used.*

30. 99288

Critical Care Services

31. 99291

> **Note:**
>
> *ED is the abbreviation for emergency department, and MDM is the abbreviation for medical decision making. The presenting problem of this patient and the fact that critical services were provided for 70 minutes requires the coding of 99291. The patient is unable to provide history due to his medical condition; however, time is the component used to assign a critical care code and the fact that the patient's medical problem is of a critical nature. The lack of history documentation does not prevent the use of code 99291 in this case.*

32. 99291, 99292, 99292, 99292, 99292

> **Note:**
>
> Three hours of critical care support equals 180 minutes, which is coded to 99291 and 99292 × 4. The criteria for critical care code assignment are the documentation of time by the physician and the patient's medical illness/condition being of a critical nature.

Nursing Facility Services

33. 99304

> **Note:**
>
> For initial nursing facility care, all three key components must be met for a specific level to be assigned. Based on the history, exam, and MDM levels in this case, 99304 is the only E/M code that can be assigned. The physician exceeds the MDM requirement for this level but does not meet the comprehensive examination requirement to be able to assign the next highest level, 99305.

34. 99308

> **Note:**
>
> For the subcategory of subsequent nursing facility care, two out of three key components must be met to assign a specific level. The exam noted in this case meets the requirement of 99308. The MDM meets the requirement of 99309. However, the case does not document that either the history or exam requirement for 99309 are met. Therefore, E/M code 99308 is assigned.

Domiciliary, Rest Home, or Custodial Care Services

35. 99324

> **Note:**
>
> The code range for domiciliary, rest home, or custodial care services is 99324 to 99328 for new patients. As with other new patient codes, three out of three key components must be met for a specific level to be assigned.

36. 99335

> **Note:**
>
> Only two out of three key components must be met for this established patient. A problem-focused history is part of level 1, an expanded problem-focused exam is part of level 2, and an MDM of moderate complexity is part of level 3. The only level where two key components were met or exceeded was level 2. The physician met the exam requirement and exceeded the MDM requirement.

Home Services

37. 99347

Note:

For the subcategory of established patient, home services, two out of three key components must be met or exceeded to assign a specific level. An MDM of a moderate level is under E/M code 99349; however, based on the level of exam and history provided, the code assigned to this case is 99347. For that code, the physician met the examination required and exceeded the MDM required. The physician also documented a problem-focused history, which is the minimal requirement for 99347. The history level and the exam level can be used to assign this code; but if the coder uses the exam and the MDM level, the E/M code is still 99347. 99348 or 99349 cannot be assigned because the documentation does not met or exceed two out of three key components. Only one (MDM) is met for either of these levels.

38. 99343

Note:

For a new patient in the category of home services, all three key components must be met or exceeded for a specific level to be assigned. For 99343, the requirements are a detailed history, a detailed examination, and MDM of moderate complexity.

Prolonged Physician Service

39. 99214, 99354, 99355

Note:

First, you have to determine the established patient office visit level based on the documentation. Then given the information of two hours of service, prolonged physician service codes are added. Based on information in CPT, 99214 has a typical time of 25 minutes. (120 minutes minus 25 minutes equals 95 minutes.) 99354 covers 74 of the 95 minutes, which leaves 21 minutes unaccounted for. 99355 is assigned for the remaining 21 minutes. Both 99354 and 99355 are add-on codes; therefore, no modifier is needed.

Physician Standby Services

40. 99360

Note:

99360 is assigned for standby (non-face-to-face) service. This code is assigned based on full units of 30 minutes.

Case Management Services

41. 99367

Note:

Code 99367 is assigned for a medical team conference of 30 minutes' duration or more with participation by the physician. Team conferences are typically face-to-face meetings of health professionals from the same discipline or from various medical specialties.

42. 99213

> ### Note:
> The patient received E/M services on the same day as the telephone service, which means the telephone is considered part of the E/M service provided. Report E/M code 99213 only.

Care Plan Oversight Services

43. 99375
44. 99378

Preventive Medicine

45. 99384

> ### Note:
> A preventive medicine service E/M code should be assigned in this case. These codes are assigned by age of the patient.

46. 99397

> ### Note:
> BPH is the abbreviation for benign prostate hypertrophy, HTN is the abbreviation for hypertension, and NIDDM is the abbreviation for non-insulin dependent diabetes mellitus. The fact that the patient is counseled on treatment options for his BPH does not preclude the assignment of a preventive medicine code. The patient came in for a check-up, which would warrant a code from this category.

Non-Face-to-Face Physician Services

47. 99441
48. 99444

Newborn Care

49. 99460 (7/8), 99238(7/9)

> ### Note:
> Code 99460 is assigned for admission, and code 99238 is assigned for normal newborn discharge service. No modifier is need because the codes are for different dates of service.

Special Evaluation and Management Services

50. 99455

> ### Note:
> Work-related or medical disability evaluation services is the subcategory of E/M codes that should be used in this case. The requirements for the assignment of an E/M from this category are the completion of a history, exam, the forming of a diagnosis, the development of a treatment plan, and the completion of a report. No special level of key components is required.

Chapter 10
CPT Anesthesia

EXERCISE 10.1 – ANESTHESIA TERMINOLOGY

1. b
2. e
3. c
4. d
5. a
6. d
7. c
8. a
9. e
10. b

EXERCISE 10.2 – OVERVIEW OF ANESTHESIA SECTION

1. Students should include five from the following list of services:

   - Draping, positioning, prepping, and transporting the patient
   - Inserting nasogastric or orogastric tubes
   - Inserting peripheral intravenous lines for fluid and medication administration
   - Interpreting laboratory results
   - Interpreting monitored functions
   - Placing airway tubes, including laryngoscopy for airway management
   - Positioning external devices for capnography, cardiac monitoring, CNS evoked responses, Doppler flow, pulse oximetry, and temperature
   - Stimulating nerves to determine level of paralysis or localization of nerve(s)

2. -59

3. False

4. Students should include three from the following list of services:

   - Monitors vital signs and maintains patient's airway and continual evaluation of vital functions
   - Diagnoses and treats clinical problems that occur during the procedure
   - Administers analgesics, anesthetic agents, hypnotics, sedatives, or other medications as necessary to ensure patient safety and comfort
   - Provides other medical services as needed for the safe completion of the procedure

5. -QS (monitored anesthesia care)

EXERCISE 10.3 – ANESTHESIA SECTION GUIDELINES

1. c
2. e
3. a
4. d
5. b
6. a
7. b
8. a
9. a
10. b
11. T
12. T
13. T
14. F
15. F
16. T
17. T
18. T
19. T
20. F

> **Note:**
>
> The anesthesia time unit is 4 because 60 ÷ 15 = 4. The anesthesia code's base unit value is 5, and the physical status modifier's relative value is 0; thus, (5 + 4 + 0) × \$17.45 = 9 × \$17.45 = \$157.05.

21. b   23. a   25. e
22. c   24. d

EXERCISE 10.4 – ANESTHESIA SUBSECTIONS

1. add-on   2. -59   3. False

> **Note:**
>
> The code description for 00326 includes the phrase, "... in children younger than 1 year of age." Therefore, code 99100 is not reported in addition to code 00326.

4. 00406   7. 00796   10. 01953
5. -QS   8. 01990
6. 01935–01936   9. 01922–23

REVIEW

Multiple Choice

1. d   8. d   15. c
2. a   9. d   16. b
3. d   10. a   17. b
4. a   11. a   18. b
5. b   12. a   19. c
6. b   13. b   20. b
7. a   14. b

Coding Practice I—Modifiers

21. 01961-P1-AA, 99140, 62318-59

> **Note:**
>
> Modifier -P1 is assigned for a healthy patient. Modifier -AA is a HCPCS modifier that is assigned to reflect anesthesia performed by an anesthesiologist. Modifier -59 is assigned to indicate that a distinct procedural service was provided in addition to anesthesia services.

22. 01832-P2-QX, 62318-59

> **Note:**
>
> CRNA is the abbreviation for certified registered nurse anesthetist. The physical status anesthesia modifier -P2 is assigned due to the patient being a diabetic. Modifier -QX is assigned to reflect CRNA service under medical direction of a physician. Modifier -59 is assigned to indicate that a distinct procedural service was provided in addition to anesthesia services.
>
> Do not report code 01996-P2-QX for monitoring on the day after surgery. That code applies to "daily hospital management of epidural or subarachnoid continuous drug administration performed after insertion of an epidural or subarachnoid catheter placed primarily for anesthesia administration during an operative session, but retained for postoperative pain management."

23. 01402-P1-AA

> **Note:**
>
> P1 is the anesthesia modifier assigned to a healthy patient, and -AA is the HCPCS modifier assigned when services are provided by an anesthesiologist.

24. 01400-P1-AA, 64447-59

> **Note:**
>
> Modifier -59 is assigned to indicate that a distinct procedural service was provided in addition to anesthesia services.

25. 00540-P2-QZ, 62318-59

> **Note:**
>
> The physical status anesthesia modifier of P2 is assigned due to this patient's chronic asthma condition. The HCPCS modifier QZ is assigned for CRNA services not under the direction of a physician. Modifier -59 is assigned to indicate that a distinct procedural service was provided in addition to anesthesia services.

Coding Practice II—Anesthesia

Head

26. 00142-P2-AA, 99100

> **Note:**
>
> The physical status anesthesia modifier of P2 is assigned due to the fact that this patient has controlled diabetes mellitus. Qualifying circumstances code 99100 is reported because the patient is over age 70.

27. 00120-P1-AA

Neck

28. 00326-P4-AA, 99100, 99140

> **Note:**
>
> *The physical status anesthesia modifier of P4 is assigned to reflect the severity of the patient's cardiopulmonary state. The qualifying circumstance code of 99100 is assigned due to the fact that the patient is less than 1 year of age. Code 99140 is reported to indicate emergency conditions of treatment.*

29. 00320-P2-AA

> **Note:**
>
> *The physical status anesthesia modifier of P2 is assigned in this case due to the nature of the patient's condition, thyroid tumor.*

Thorax (Chest Wall and Shoulder Girdle)

30. 00400-P1-AA
31. 00474-P2-AA

> **Note:**
>
> *The patient's chest pain, shortness of breath, and possible lordosis are symptoms of pectus excavatum. While most patients with pectus excavatum are asymptomatic, this patient exhibited symptoms that interfered with physiologic functioning. Therefore, the physical status modifier is -P2. (If the patient had remained untreated and his symptoms had worsened, resulting in heart and/or respiratory disease, physical status modifier -P3 would have been assigned.)*

Intrathoracic

32. 00524-P3-AA, 99100

> **Note:**
>
> *The qualifying circumstance code of 99100 is assigned due to the patient's age being over 70. The physical status anesthesia modifier -P3 is assigned for the systemic disease of pneumonia and the severity that caused the patient to have drainage of fluid (pneumocentesis).*

33. 00530-P2-AA

Spine and Spinal Cord

34. 00600-P2-AA
35. 00635-P2-AA

Upper Abdomen

36. 00756-P2-AA
37. 00702-P1-AA

Lower Abdomen

38. 00802-P1-AA

> **Note:**
>
> *This patient has no medical history or chronic conditions; therefore, the physical status anesthesia modifier -P1 is assigned.*

39. 00851-P1-AA

Perineum

40. 00952-P2-AA
41. 00921-P1-AA

Pelvis

42. 01112-P1-AA
43. 01170-P1-AA

Upper Leg

44. 01230-P2-AA

> **Note:**
>
> *Type 2 diabetes mellitus is a systemic disease that is under control in this patient. Therefore, the physical status modifier -P2 is assigned.*

45. 01214-P3-AA, 99100

> **Note:**
>
> *The physical status modifier -P3 is assigned due to the admitted condition of the patient.*

Knee and Popliteal Area

46. 01392-P1-AA
47. 01400-P1-AA

Lower Leg

48. 01462-P2-AA

> **Note:**
>
> *The physical status modifier -P2 is assigned in this case due to the patient's preexisting condition of Down syndrome.*

49. 01462-P1-AA

> **Note:**
>
> *The fact that this patient is a smoker does not warrant a higher-level physical status modifier. There is no documentation of any disease process or condition; therefore, modifier -P1 is assigned.*

Shoulder and Axilla

50. 01620-P1-AA

51. 01636-P1-AA

Upper Arm and Elbow

52. 01710-P1-AA

53. 01716-P1-AA

Forearm, Wrist, and Hand

54. 01810-P1-AA

55. 01830-P1-AA

Radiologic Procedures

56. 01920-P2-AA

57. 01922-P3-AA

Burn Excisions or Debridement

58. 01952-P3-AA, 01953, 01953, 01953

> **Note:**
>
> *01952 covers 9 percent of this patient's 35 percent total body burn. Thirty-five percent minus 9 percent equals 26 percent (35 − 9 = 26). 01953 is added × 3 to reflect the remaining 26 percent. 01953 is an add-on code; therefore, no -51 modifier is required.*

59. 01952-P2-AA

Obstetric

60. 01960-P1-AA

61. 01961-P2-AA

Other Procedures

62. 01996-P1-AA

63. 01990-P6-AA

64. 96365

> **Note:**
>
> *Do not report Modifiers -P1 or -AA with code 96365.*

65. 00172-P2-AA, 99100

> **Note:**
>
> *Modifier -P2 is added due to the diagnosis of cleft palate. Qualifying code of 99100 is assigned because the child is under the age of 1 year.*

Chapter 11
CPT Surgery I

EXERCISE 11.1 – OVERVIEW OF SURGERY SECTION

1. body area or organ system

2. diagnostic

3. therapeutic

4. a. urinary system
   b. urinary bladder
   c. endoscopic
   d. biopsy
   e. cystourethroscopy with biopsy
   f. 52204

> **Note:**
>
> Combination code 52204 includes cystourethroscopy with biopsy. No incision is made to access the urinary bladder because the cystourethroscope is inserted through the urethra into the urinary bladder.

5. a. digestive system
   b. large intestine (colon)
   c. laparotomy (incision)
   d. excision
   e. partial colon resection (colectomy) with anastomosis
   f. 44140

> **Note:**
>
> Do not code the lysis of adhesions or exploratory laparotomy. The lysis of adhesions is incidental to the colon resection procedure, and the exploratory laparotomy is the surgical approach. To find the code, refer to the CPT index and locate main term Colon, subterm Excision, and 2nd qualifier Partial. Review the range of codes to select 44140 (Colectomy, partial; with anastomosis). (Since there is no mention of laparoscopic approach in the case study, do not report code 44204.)

EXERCISE 11.2 – SURGERY GUIDELINES

1. F	4. F	7. T
2. T	5. F	
3. T	6. T	

> ### Note:
>
> *When a diagnostic procedure (e.g., diagnostic esophagogastroduodenoscopy) is performed and the provider performs follow-up evaluation and management (E/M) services, the E/M service(s) are separately coded and reported. (If the patient had undergone a therapeutic procedure, such as a partial gastrectomy to remove that part of the stomach that had ulcers, and the physician provided follow-up E/M services, a separate code would not be reported. Such follow-up E/M services are part of the global period and, therefore, included in the procedure code that was initially reported.)*

8. F
9. T
10. T

11. July 30
12. March 15
13. October 14

14. -24

15. Although code 29870 contains "(separate procedure)" in its description, that procedure was performed separately and independently of the related and more comprehensive procedure performed the next day. In addition, the first procedure was diagnostic and the second procedure was performed to repair the knee.

16. -50

17. Typically a biopsy of the vulva or perineum is not performed during the same operative session as an inguinal hernia repair. The biopsy is unrelated to the repair of the inguinal hernia. Therefore, modifier -59 is added to code 56605 to indicate that the biopsy was unrelated to the repair of the inguinal hernia.

18. 29999 (Unlisted procedure, arthroscopy)

19. Ablation of benign, premalignant, or malignant tissues by any method, with or without curettement, including local anesthesia, and not usually requiring closure

20. Once because the description states "15 or more lesions." (Also, do *not* report modifier -51 with code 17004.)

EXERCISE 11.3 – GENERAL SUBSECTION

1. 10021

2. 10022
   76942

EXERCISE 11.4 – INCISION AND DRAINAGE

1. 10180
2. 10140

3. 10120
4. 10040

5. 10061

EXERCISE 11.5 – LESION REMOVAL

1. 11401

> ### Note:
>
> *Do not report modifier -LT with CPT integumentary system codes because the skin is not a paired organ. The procedure in #1, above, was performed on the "skin" of the left forearm.*

2. 11000, 11001
3. 11643, 11602–51, 11602–51

4. 11056
5. 11442

EXERCISE 11.6 – NAILS

1. 11719-TA, 11719-T1, 11719-T2, 11719-T3, 11719-T4, 11719-T5, 11719-T6, 11719-T7, 11719-T8, 11719-T9

Note:

- Do not add modifier -50 to the code because the code description includes the phrase *any number*.
- Report code 11719 × 10, with the appropriate modifier attached to each (to indicate that all ten toes were treated).

2. 11762-T1
3. 11730-T5, 11732-T6, 11732-T7, 11732-T8, 11732-T9
4. 11740-F1
5. 11765-T7

EXERCISE 11.7 – PILONIDAL CYST

1. 11772
2. 11770
3. 11771
4. 10080
5. 10081

EXERCISE 11.8 – INTRODUCTION

1. 11980
2. 11900
3. 11954
4. 11976
5. 11901

EXERCISE 11.9 – REPAIR (CLOSURE)

1. 12002
2. Report an appropriate E/M code because there is no CPT surgery code for a wound closure with adhesive strips.
3. 16020
4. 15200, 15002
5. 15780

EXERCISE 11.10 – DESTRUCTION

1. 17000, 17003 x 2

Note:

Report code 17003 twice because of the word *each* in the CPT code description.

2. 11200, 11201

Note:

Report code 11201 in addition to 11200 because a total of 17 skin tags were removed. Code 11200 is reported for the first 15 skin tags removed, and code 11201 is reported for up to the next 10 skin tags removed.

3. 17110
4. 17000, 17003
5. 11200

6. 17274
7. 17262
8. 17276

9. 17280
10. 17263-LT

EXERCISE 11.11 - BREAST

1. 19125-RT, 19126-RT
2. 19367-RT

3. 19301-LT
4. 19302-RT

5. 19102-LT, 19295-LT, 77032

REVIEW

Multiple Choice

1. d
2. b
3. a
4. d
5. c
6. b

7. b
8. c
9. c
10. a
11. c
12. c

13. c
14. b
15. b
16. d
17. b

> **Note:**
>
> Modifier -LT is not added to any codes in this question because the surgery was performed on skin, which is not considered a paired organ.

18. d

19. a

20. d

Coding Practice

General

21. 10021

22. 10022, 77012

Integumentary System

23. 11404

24. 11771

> **Note:**
>
> Code 11771 is reported for extensive excision of a pilonidal cyst, which is one that is over 2 cm in size, is recurrent, and/or requires subcutaneous or layer closure. For this case, a 5.0 cm pilonidal subcutaneous cyst was removed and layered closure was required.

25. 10060

26. 15100, 11606

> **Note:**
>
> Do not report modifier -LT for general skin procedures because the skin is not considered a paired organ.

27. 13132-F1

> **Note:**
>
> For this case, surgical debridement and depth of the repair indicates the complex closure of a traumatic laceration.

28. 16020

> **Note:**
>
> Do not report code 11040, which describes partial-thickness skin debridement. Code 16020 specifically classifies a procedure performed for treatment of a burn, and it includes partial-thickness skin debridement.

29. 11730-T5, 11732-TA

> **Note:**
>
> Code 11730 is assigned for removal (or avulsion) of one nail plate, and code 11732 is assigned for removal of the second nail plate of the left great toe. HCPCS level II modifiers are added to the codes to indicate the digits on which the procedures were performed. (-T5 is added to indicate surgery on the right foot, great toe. -TA is added to indicate surgery on the left foot, great toe.)

30. 12002

> **Note:**
>
> Per CPT notes, wound repairs of the same anatomical group and same level of repair have lengths added together to determine the code assignment. In this case, the lengths of the neck and scalp wounds are totaled. (3.0 + 2.0 = 5.0 cm.) Both repairs are simple, and the correct code is 12002. (Do not assign codes 12002 and 12001.)

31. 15740   32. 15840

> **Note:**
>
> Obtaining the fascial graft is included in code 15840. Do not report a separate code for obtaining the graft.

33. 17273

> **Note:**
>
> Surgical curettement is a type of destruction, and a code from range 17000–17286 is assigned.

34. 19301-LT   35. 19000-RT

Chapter 12
CPT Surgery II

EXERCISE 12.1 – MUSCULOSKELETAL SYSTEM NOTES

1. body area
2. open or closed fractures and joint injuries
3. treatment
4. normal, uncomplicated follow-up care
5. manipulation

EXERCISE 12.2 – GENERAL

1. 20000   2. 20005   3. 20101

> **Note:**
>
> Surgical exploration and enlargement of the wound, debridement removal of a foreign body, and ligation of subcutaneous tissue is included in 20101; do not report separate codes.

4. 20240

> **Note:**
>
> Even though this procedure was performed on the left femur, do not add modifier -LT to code 20240. Its code description does not represent a procedure performed on paired organs because the sternum and spinous process is listed as an example.

5. 20612-RT   6. 20692

> **Note:**
>
> Do not add modifier -RT to code 20692. Its code description does not represent a procedure performed on paired organs.

7. 20816-F6

> **Note:**
>
> Do not report modifier -LT. Modifier -F6 specifies the right second (index) finger. MCP is the abbreviation for metacarpophalangeal (joint).

8. 20920   9. 20931   10. 20975

EXERCISE 12.3 – HEAD

1. 21010-50   2. 21026

> **Note:**
>
> Report code 21026 just once because the code description includes the term bone(s).

3. 21084   5. 21150   7. 21270
4. 21121   6. 21198   8. 21401

> **Note:**
>
> There is no mention of the term blowout; therefore, do not report a code from 21385–21395.

9. 21440   10. 21465

EXERCISE 12.4 – NECK (SOFT TISSUES), THORAX, BACK, AND FLANK

1. 21510   3. 21820   5. 21627
2. 21685   4. 21600   6. 20206

> **Note:**
>
> The parenthetical note below code 21550 provides instruction to report code 20206 for a needle biopsy of (any) soft tissue.

7. 21930   8. 21935

> **Note:**
>
> A radical resection includes excision of the tumor; therefore, do not report code 21930 in addition to code 21935.

9. 21920   10. 21925

EXERCISE 12.5 – SPINE (VERTEBRAL COLUMN)

1. 22630

> **Note:**
>
> Just one interspace was fused; therefore, report code 22630. Also, code 22630 includes laminectomy and diskectomy when performed to prepare the vertebral interspace for fusion.

2. 22505

> **Note:**
>
> Report code 22505 just once even though three spinal regions were manipulated under anesthesia.

3. 22220   4. 22841   5. 22800, 20937

EXERCISE 12.6 – ABDOMEN, SHOULDER, HUMERUS (UPPER ARM) AND ELBOW, FOREARM AND WRIST, AND HAND AND FINGERS

1. 22900
2. 23000-LT
3. 23900-RT

> **Note:**
>
> An interthoracoscapular amputation (forequarter) is the surgical amputation of the arm, including disarticulation (separation at the joint) of the humerus and removal of the scapula and outer part of the clavicle (collarbone).

4. 23331-LT
5. 24075-RT
6. 24357-RT
7. 24300-LT
8. 25606-LT
9. 25246-RT
10. 26121-LT

EXERCISE 12.7 – PELVIS AND HIP JOINT, FEMUR (THIGH REGION) AND KNEE JOINT, LEG (TIBIA AND FIBULA) AND ANKLE JOINT, AND FOOT AND TOES

1. 27097
2. 27125-RT

> **Note:**
>
> If the patient returns in the future for replacement of the prosthetic device (e.g., broken device), report code 27236.

3. 27372-LT
4. 27323-LT
5. 27357-LT

> **Note:**
>
> Code 27357 includes obtaining (harvesting) graft, such as femur tissue, when performed during the same operative episode.

6. 27498-RT
7. 27650-RT
8. 27604-LT
9. 28296-RT
10. 28110-RT

EXERCISE 12.8 – APPLICATION OF CASTS AND STRAPPING AND ENDOSCOPY/ARTHROSCOPY

1. 29830-LT
2. 29065-LT

> **Note:**
>
> Do not report code 29705-LT because the same physician who applied the first cast removed the wet cast and applied the new cast.

3. 29086-F9

> **Note:**
>
> The proximal interphalangeal (PIP) joint is part of the finger. Therefore, add modifier -F9 (not -RT) to the code.

4. 29445-LT	7. 29901-RT	10. 29881-LT
5. 29125-LT	8. 29824-LT	
6. 29892-RT	9. 29807-RT	

EXERCISE 12.9 – NOSE

1. 30200

> **Note:**
>
> Do not add modifier -50 to code 30200 because its description indicates turbinate(s), indicating surgery performed on multiple and bilateral turbinates.

2. 30110-LT

> **Note:**
>
> Do not report a code for single-layer closure, which is a simple closure that is included with code 30110.

3. 30100-LT   4. 30118-LT

> **Note:**
>
> The CPT index entry for "Rhinotomy, lateral" lists code 30118 and 30320. No foreign body was removed; therefore, report code 30118 with the appropriate directional modifier.

5. 30462

EXERCISE 12.10 – ACCESSORY SINUSES

1. 31200	3. 31255-LT, 31256-51-LT	5. 31276-LT
2. 31238	4. 31237	

> **Note:**
>
> Do not report a code for diagnostic endoscopy (31231) because it is included in the surgical endoscopy code.

EXERCISE 12.11 – LARYNX

1. 31500	3. 31587	5. 31365, 38720-59
2. 31365	4. 31502	

Note:

- *For a total laryngectomy with bilateral radical neck dissection (31365), do not add modifier -50 to the code. The larynx is a single midline organ, and it is not appropriate to add modifier -50 to code 31365. (A laryngectomy cannot be performed bilaterally.)*
- *Instead, report code 31365 for the total laryngectomy and radical neck dissection on one side. Then, report code 38720-59 for the radical neck dissection on the other side (even though the description of code 38720 is "Cervical lymphadenectomy (complete)."*
- *Add modifier -59 to indicate a distinct procedural service.*

EXERCISE 12.12 – TRACHEA AND BRONCHI

1. 31603   2. 31717

Note:

Do not report code 31700 because that procedure is included in the description of code 31717. The description of code 31700 contains the phrase (separate procedure).

3. 31635-LT   4. 31624   5. 31623, 31625, 31635

Note:

Codes 31623, 31625, and 31635 are distinct surgical procedures, and they are not considered integral components of one another. Therefore, report each code separately and do not add modifier -51 to any of the codes.

EXERCISE 12.13 – LUNGS AND PLEURA

1. 32551   3. 32405, 10021
2. 32997   4. 32663

Note:

Do not report code 32601 because diagnostic thoracoscopy is included in the code for surgical thoracoscopy.

5. 32851, 32850, 35216, 32855

REVIEW

Multiple Choice

1. b   4. c   7. a
2. a   5. d   8. d
3. b   6. d

> **Note:**
>
> C3-C4 contains just one interspace; therefore, report code 22554 just once (with modifier -62 added to indicate that two surgeons were required to perform the procedure).

9. d	13. b	17. c
10. c	14. a	18. a
11. c	15. d	19. c
12. c	16. c	20. d

Coding Practice

Musculoskeletal System

21. 20100

> **Note:**
>
> Codes 20100–20103 are reported for wound exploration resulting from penetrating trauma (e.g., penetrating gunshot or stab wound). These codes include surgical exploration, extension of dissection, debridement, removal of foreign bodies, and ligation/coagulation of minor subcutaneous/muscular blood vessels (not requiring thoracotomy or laparotomy). Do not report simple, intermediate, or complex repair (closure) codes from the Integumentary subsection with a wound exploration (trauma) code.

22. 21179

> **Note:**
>
> Do not report a separate code for the bone allograft.

23. 27506-RT

> **Note:**
>
> Do not report a separate code for placement of the splint. The splint application is included in the code for the open fracture treatment.

24. 27301-RT   25. 27570-LT   26. 29345-LT

> **Note:**
>
> For cast reapplication, assign a code from 29000–29799. Do not code the cast removal. Cast removal is coded only when performed by a different physician.

27. 29730-LT   28. 29830-LT   29. 26080-F6

> **Note:**
>
> The incision was made between the first and second bones of the right index finger, which is an interphalangeal joint. Code 26080 is assigned. (Do not mistakenly assign code 26075, which involves surgery on the metacarpophalangeal joint, which is located between the first bone of the finger and bones of the wrist.)

30. 25600-RT

> **Note:**
> Do not report a separate code for application of the cast. The cast application is included in the code for the open fracture treatment.

Respiratory System

31. 31231

> **Note:**
> Do not add modifier -50 to the code. The code descriptor states that this code is applied to unilateral or bilateral procedures. There is no need to apply the -50 modifier.

32. 31510

> **Note:**
> An indirect laryngoscopy uses a mirror to visualize the larynx.

33. 31576   34. 32656

> **Note:**
> The insertion of a chest tube is a common component of this procedure and is not separately coded.

35. 31628   36. 31561

> **Note:**
> Do not report a separate code for use of the operating microscope (69990).

37. 30520   39. 30300
38. 30100   40. 30460

Chapter 13
CPT Surgery III

EXERCISE 13.1 – HEART AND PERICARDIUM

1. 33410
2. 33824
3. 33533, 33517

> **Note:**
> Do not report modifier -51 with code 33517.

4. 33920
5. 33208, 33225

> **Note:**
> Do not report modifier -51 with code 33225.

6. 33031
7. 33282, 93285
8. 33702
9. 33261
10. 33922
11. 33010, 76930
12. 33215
13. 33250
14. 33510, 33508
15. 33690
16. 33464
17. 33496
18. 33512
19. 33533, 33572
20. 33606
21. 33641

> **Note:**
> Do not report separate codes for the cardiopulmonary bypass or patch. Code 33641 includes repair of the defect, cardiopulmonary bypass, and placement of the patch.

22. 33852
23. 33780
24. 33641
25. 33860

EXERCISE 13.2 – ARTERIES AND VEINS

1. 37202

> **Note:**
> NCCI edits allow the reporting of code 37202 with the cardiac catheterization code.

2. 75710, 36120
3. 36200, 75605, 75625
4. 36555
5. 36011-LT, 36012-LT, 75831-LT

EXERCISE 13.3 – HEMIC AND LYMPHATIC SYSTEMS SUBSECTION

1. 38572
2. 38204
3. 38242
4. 38208
5. 38221
6. 38207
7. 38100
8. 38115
9. 38200, 75810
10. 38100
11. 38120
12. 38700
13. 41155, 38724-59

Note:

When a cervical lymphadenectomy (38720–38724) is performed during the same operative session as a bilateral neck resection or dissection, report code 41155 for the cervical lymphadenectomy and resection on side. Report code 38724 with the appropriate modifier for the modified neck dissection performed on the other side. (Do not report directional modifiers -LT and -RT because each side of the neck is not considered a paired organ.)

14. 31365, 38720-59

Note:

When a total laryngectomy with bilateral radical neck dissection (31365) is performed, code 31365 is reported for the total laryngectomy and radical neck dissection on one side. (There is just one larynx, which means that modifier -50 cannot be added to code 31365.) Code 38720-59 is reported for the radical neck dissection on the other side. (Modifier -59 is added to indicate a distinct procedural service.) (Do not report directional modifiers -LT and -RT because each side of the neck is not considered a paired organ.)

15. 38792, 78195

REVIEW

Multiple Choice

1. d
2. a
3. c
4. d
5. d
6. b
7. b
8. d
9. c
10. d
11. c
12. d
13. b
14. b
15. c
16. b
17. d
18. d
19. c
20. c

Coding Practice

Cardiovascular System

21. 37722-50, 37718-51-LT

Note:

The patient had bilateral long saphenous vein stripping, which is reflected with CPT code 37722; modifier -50 identifies this as a bilateral procedure. The patient had short veins stripped of the left leg. Modifier -51 is added to code 37718 to reflect multiple procedures reported on the same date of service. HCPCS modifier -LT is added to reflect that the procedure of stripping short veins was done on the left side of the patient's body.

22. 33430   23. 33208

> **Note:**
>
> *33208 includes insertion of the pulse generator and electrodes into the atrial and ventricular areas.*

24. 33820   26. 36830   27. 35301-LT
25. 36425

> **Note:**
>
> *EEG is the abbreviation for electroencephalogram. The EEG done during the operation is a common component of this procedure and is not separately coded or reported. To do so would be unbundling.*

28. 33241, 33240-78

> **Note:**
>
> *This case documents the insertion of a new pulse generator only. The leads were not replaced.*

29. 32140   30. 33510

Hemic and Lymphatic Systems
31. 38221   34. 38770   37. 38790, 75805
32. 38100   35. 38520
33. 38555   36. 38120

> **Note:**
>
> *Code 38790 is reported for the injection, and code 75805 is reported for the radiologic procedure.*

38. 38382

> **Note:**
>
> *Chyle in the pleural cavity is a condition called chylothorax.*

39. 38204   40. 38300

Chapter 14
CPT Surgery IV

EXERCISE 14.1 – MEDIASTINUM AND DIAPHRAGM SUBSECTION

1. 39561
2. 39010
3. 39502
4. 39400
5. 39540

EXERCISE 14.2 – ORAL CAVITY

1. 41874
2. 40500
3. 40810
4. 41010

> **Note:**
>
> Do not report code 40819, which classifies an excision of the frenum.

5. 42330

> **Note:**
>
> Do not report code 42405, which classifies an incisional biopsy.

6. 42953
7. 42700
8. 42820
9. 42960
10. 42826

> **Note:**
>
> Do not report code 42821, which classifies a tonsillectomy and adenoidectomy. This patient underwent tonsillectomy only.

EXERCISE 14.3 – ESOPHAGUS AND STOMACH

1. 43217
2. 43045

> **Note:**
>
> Do not report code 43101, which classifies excision of a lesion from the esophagus. This patient underwent foreign body removal from the esophagus through an incision in the chest wall and esophagus (esophagotomy).

3. 43460
4. 43116-52-62 (Dr. Smith), 43496-62 (Dr. Jones)
5. 43250,43251-59

6. 43520

7. 43848

8. 43761, 75984

> **Note:**
>
> Do not report code 43752, which classifies the original placement of a nasogastric or orogastric tube. Because fluoroscopic guidance is not included in code 43761, report code 75984.

9. 43644

> **Note:**
>
> Do not report code 43645, which classifies small intestine reconstruction to limit absorption in addition to the gastric bypass procedure.

10. 49440

EXERCISE 14.4 – INTESTINES (EXCEPT RECTUM), MECKEL'S DIVERTICULUM AND THE MESENTERY, APPENDIX, RECTUM, AND ANUS

1. 44955 (in addition to cesarean section code)

2. 44005

3. 44120, 44121

> **Note:**
>
> Two segments of small intestine were resected and anastomosed. Therefore, report primary code 44120 and add-on code 44121. Do not report code 44625, which classifies the closure of an enterostomy with resection and anastomosis.

4. 44850	6. 45000	7. 45114
5. 44206		

> **Note:**
>
> Do not report code 45135, which classifies an excision of rectal procidentia, with anastomosis, abdominal and perineal approach.

8. 45300	9. 45333	10. 45384

EXERCISE 14.5 – LIVER; BILIARY TRACT; PANCREAS; AND ABDOMEN, PERITONEUM, AND OMENTUM

1. 47011	2. 47141	3. 47380

> **Note:**
>
> Do not report code 47370, which is performed via laparoscopy. The procedure for this case was performed via open laparotomy.

4. 47564

> **Note:**
>
> Do not report code 47610, which is performed via open incision (not laparoscopy).

5. 47480   7. 49002   8. 49650
6. 49081

> **Note:**
>
> Do not report a code for use of the mesh. (A code for the use of mesh is reported for incisional or ventral hernia repair only.)

9. 49560, 49568   10. 49495

> **Note:**
>
> Do not report code 49496, which classifies an incarcerated or strangulated hernia.

EXERCISE 14.6 – URINARY SYSTEM SUBSECTION

1. 50020
2. 50590-LT
3. 50060-RT
4. 50392-RT, 74475-RT

5. 50542-LT
6. 50600-LT
7. 50953-50
8. 50727-RT

9. 50684-LT, 74425-LT
10. 50605-LT
11. 52500

> **Note:**
>
> Do not report code 52640, which is performed for a postoperative bladder neck contracture.

12. 52325   13. 52700   14. 51102

> **Note:**
>
> Do not report code 51045, which classifies a cystotomy (incision made into the urinary bladder) with insertion of ureteral catheter or stent.

15. 52214, 52320-51   17. 53600   19. 53850
16. 53440   18. 53400   20. 53200

REVIEW

Multiple Choice

1. b	8. a	15. a
2. b	9. a	16. b
3. a	10. c	17. c
4. d	11. b	18. a
5. c	12. d	19. b
6. d	13. c	20. c
7. b	14. b	

Coding Practice

Mediastinum and Diaphragm

21. 39200

> **Note:**
>
> *MRI is the abbreviation for magnetic resonance imaging.*

22. 39540
23. 39545

> **Note:**
>
> *Imbrication is the overlapping of diaphragm tissue.*

24. 39501	25. 39400

Digestive System

26. 43840	30. 49553	34. 41015
27. 40510	31. 47562	35. 42410
28. 43611	32. 45331	
29. 42821	33. 47100	

> **Note:**
>
> *Do not report code 42415 because there is no documentation of "nerve dissection." The mass was dissected free; however, the facial nerve was not dissected.*

Urinary System

36. 52214	38. 52235	40. 50590-RT
37. 52310	39. 50021	41. 52332-RT

> **Note:**
>
> *Do not report code 52000-LT in addition to 52332-RT even though the cystourethroscope was also passed into the left ureter to visualize it. Because the cystourethroscope had already been passed through the urethra to visualize the right ureter (and to facilitate inserting the double-J stent), third-party payers will not consider passing the cystourethroscope into the left ureter a separate procedure. (After using the cystourethroscope to insert the double-J stent), the surgeon withdraws the instrument from the right ureter and inserts it into the left ureter. The instrument did not have to be completely withdrawn from the urethra and reinserted through the urethral to then visualize the left ureter.)*

42. 51535

43. 50200-RT

44. 50060-RT

45. 53400

Chapter 15
CPT Surgery V

EXERCISE 15.1 – MALE GENITAL SYSTEM SUBSECTION

1. 55150   2. 55520-LT   3. 54550-RT

> **Note:**
>
> Do not report code 55110, which classifies scrotal exploration.

4. 55812   5. 54050

EXERCISE 15.2 – INTERSEX SURGERY SUBSECTION

1. 55970   2. 55980

EXERCISE 15.3 – FEMALE GENITAL SYSTEM SUBSECTION

1. 58605 (in addition to vaginal delivery code)
2. 57020

> **Note:**
>
> Colpocentesis involves making an incision in the vaginal wall to drain peritoneal fluid from the area behind the vagina. This case did not mention the presence of a peritoneal abscess; therefore, do not report code 57010.

3. 58970   4. 58300   5. 58662

EXERCISE 15.4 – MATERNITY CARE AND DELIVERY SUBSECTION

1. 59120   3. 59012, 76941   5. 59426, 59430
2. 59000, 76946   4. 59025

EXERCISE 15.5 – ENDOCRINE SYSTEM SUBSECTION

1. 60300   2. 60225

> ### Note:
>
> - The total thyroid lobectomy was performed on the right, which means it's a unilateral total thyroid lobectomy. A contralateral subtotal lobectomy including isthmusectomy was also performed during the same operative episode, which means it was performed on the left side. Thus, code 60225 is assigned because it states, "Total thyroid lobectomy, unilateral; with contralateral subtotal lobectomy, including isthmusectomy."
> - Do not assign modifiers to code 60225.
> - Do not assign code 60220 in addition to code 60225 because that would be considered overcoding. Code 60225 includes all elements of the procedure performed.

3. 60260   5. 60000   7. 60500, 60512
4. 60100   6. 60540

> ### Note:
>
> The parenthetical note below code 60512 instructs the coder to report that code with 60500, 60502, 60505, 60212, 60225, 60240, 60252, 60254, 60260, 60270, and 60271.

8. 60540   9. 60500   10. 60600

EXERCISE 15.6 – NERVOUS SYSTEM SUBSECTION

1. 61305

> ### Note:
>
> Per the parenthetical note below code 61253 in CPT, do not report code 61253 with code 61305 when burr holes are drilled into the infratentorial area prior to craniectomy during the same operative session.

2. 61210   5. 61070   8. 63740
3. 61215   6. 63012   9. 62361
4. 62252   7. 62270   10. 63064

> ### Note:
>
> T-1 represents one thoracic vertebral segment. Therefore, code 63064 is reported. If more than one thoracic vertebral segment was decompressed, code 63066 would be reported for each additional segment.

11. 64410   13. 64420   15. 64550
12. 64475-50, 64476-50   14. 64786

EXERCISE 15.7 – EYE AND OCULAR ADNEXA SUBSECTION

1. 65222-RT   4. 65265-RT   7. 65820-RT, 66990-RT
2. 65275-LT   5. 65205-E3
3. 65125   6. 65450-LT

> **Note:**
>
> *Report add-on code 66990 as an additional code to indicate the use of an ophthalmic endoscope during the goniotomy procedure.*

8. 66985-58-RT

> **Note:**
>
> *Modifier -58 indicates that a staged or related procedure was performed.*

9. 65400-LT   11. 67015-RT   13. 67227-50
10. 66984-LT   12. 67220-RT, 92235-RT

> **Note:**
>
> *Do not report code 67101, which classifies repair of retinal detachment.*

14. 67255-LT   17. 67312-50   20. 67312-RT, 67320-RT
15. 67141-LT   18. 67805-E1–E3
16. 67415-RT   19. 67311-RT, 67318-LT

> **Note:**
>
> *Report code 67320 just once because its description does not specify "each" muscle.*

21. 68200-LT   22. 68761-50, 68761-50

> **Note:**
>
> - *There are four puncta, two associated with each eye. Code 68761-50 classifies surgery performed on two puncta (one associated with each eye). Reporting code 68761-50 twice classifies surgery performed on four puncta (two associated with each eye).*
> - *Medicare coding guidelines state that code 68761 is reported four times (instead of using modifier -50).*

23. 68810-50   24. 68705-LT, 68705-LT

> **Note:**
>
> *Two puncta are associated with each eye. Therefore, report code 68705-LT twice to classify surgery performed on two puncta of one eye.*

25. 68020-RT

EXERCISE 15.8 – AUDITORY SYSTEM SUBSECTION

1. 69000-LT
2. 69200-LT
3. 69300-RT
4. 69220-RT
5. 69090-50
6. 69424-50
7. 69436-50
8. 69405-50
9. 69710-LT
10. 69650-LT
11. 69720
12. 69930-50
13. 69610-RT
14. 69642-LT
15. 69676-LT
16. 69970-LT
17. 69955
18. 69960-RT
19. 69970
20. 69950

EXERCISE 15.9 – OPERATING MICROSCOPE SUBSECTION

1. 69610

> **Note:**
>
> *Operating Microscope notes state that code 69990 are not reported for visualization with magnifying loupe or corrected vision.*

2. 31526

> **Note:**
>
> *The description for code 31526 states "with operating microscope," which means that code 69990 is not reported separately.*

3. 19301-RT, 69990   4. 54901, 69990   5. 61548

> **Note:**
>
> *Do not add code 69990 because below code 61548 is a parenthetical note that states, "(Do not report code 69990 in addition to code 61548.)"*

REVIEW

Multiple Choice

1. d	8. b	15. b
2. b	9. d	16. d
3. b	10. c	17. d
4. c	11. c	18. c
5. a	12. d	19. b
6. a	13. a	20. b
7. d	14. b	

CODING PRACTICE

Male Genital System

21. 55700   22. 55041

> **Note:**
>
> The code description for 55041 states that it is a bilateral code. Do not add modifier -50 to the code.

23. 54057	26. 55250	29. 54840
24. 54150	27. 55815	30. 54300
25. 54522-50	28. 54600-LT	

Female Genital System

31. 58240

> **Note:**
>
> Due to this patient's diagnosis of gynecologic malignancy, the code assignment is different than that of a non-gynecologic abdominal hysterectomy (58150). Also, this patient had a pelvic exenteration, or removal, of the contents of the cavity.

32. 58558	35. 57135	38. 58770
33. 58671	36. 56740	39 58974
34. 57454	37. 57513	40 58925

Intersex Surgery

41. 55980   42. 55970

Maternity Care and Delivery

43. 59050

Note:

Fetal monitoring during labor by the attending obstetrician is not a separately billable or reportable service. The service done in this case is performed by a specialist, or neonatologist, which is billable and reportable per CPT guidelines.

44. 59618

Note:

This patient requested a VBAC (vaginal birth after cesarean). However, due to fetal distress, this request could not be granted; and the mother had a repeat c-section. Attempted VBAC that is unsuccessful is reported with 59618, not 59610. 59610 is the code used to report a successful VBAC.

45. 59866   47. 59414   49. 59400
46. 59812   48. 59120

Note:

Per CPT guidelines, the performing of an episiotomy during a delivery is not a separately billable or reportable procedure. To do so is unbundling. This code also reflects antepartum and postpartum care.

50. 59425   51. 59400, 59412

Note:

CPT code 59400 reflects normal antepartum care, vaginal delivery, and routine postpartum care. CPT code 59412 reflects the turning of the fetus from a breech presentation to a cephalic presentation. Modifier -51 is added to reflect multiple procedure codes being reported.

Endocrine System

52. 60100   55. 60281   58. 60220
53. 60220   56. 60500   59. 60254
54. 60540-50   57. 60650-LT

Note:

The patient has a thyroid malignancy, which requires the assignment of code 60254 for a total excision, not code 60240.

60. 60260   61. 60545-LT

Nervous System

62. 62360   63. 64402

> **Note:**
>
> A nerve block is the terminology used to identify the injection of an anesthetic agent into a nerve.

64. 64831-LT   66. 63700   68. 61150
65. 64553   67. 62270   69. 61680

> **Note:**
>
> AV is the abbreviation for arteriovenous.

70. 64712   71. 63744

Eye and Ocular Adnexa System

72. 65222-LT   73. 67312-LT

> **Note:**
>
> Each eye has four extraocular muscles: superior rectus, inferior rectus, lateral rectus, and medial rectus. In this case, two muscles were surgically treated.

74. 67800-E1   77. 66761-LT   80. 68550-LT
75. 68520-RT   78. 67145-RT   81. 66984-LT
76. 65400-RT   79. 67938-E4

> **Note:**
>
> - IOL is the abbreviation for intraocular lens.
> - The use of the operating microscope is included in the code because it is an integral part of cataract surgery. Assigning a separate code for use of an operating microscope (69990) in addition to the code for the eye surgery is unbundling.
> - The injection of an antibiotic is considered an integral part of the procedure, and a separate code is not assigned.

Auditory System

82. 69210

> **Note:**
>
> Modifier -50 is not added to the code for this case. The description of code 69210 indicates that this code is reportable for unilateral or bilateral procedures.

83. 69300-LT   85. 69105-RT   86. 69636-LT
84. 69200-LT

Note:

The removal of the cholesteatoma is an incidental part of this procedure, and it is not separately coded.

87. 69540-LT   89. 69400-RT
88. 69020-RT   90. 69552-LT

Note:

The tegmen is part of the mastoid bone; it is the roof the mastoid sinuses.

91. 69220-LT

Operating Microscope

Note:

Code 69990 for use of the operating microscope is an add-on code. Do not add modifier -51 to the code.

92. 69801-RT, 69990   96. 26548-F4, 69990   100. 31420, 69990
93. 42600-LT, 69990   97. 35207-F3, 69990   101. 26415-LT, 69990
94. 39503, 69990   98. 64865, 69990   102. 69424-50, 69990
95. 34501-LT, 69990   99. 42808, 69990

Note:

Modifier -50 is added to the procedure code to reflect that it is a bilateral procedure.

103. 51500, 69990   104. 26483-F6, 69990   105. 24495, 69990

Chapter 16
CPT Radiology

EXERCISE 16.1 – RADIOLOGY TERMINOLOGY

1. d	6. d	11. d
2. a	7. a	12. e
3. c	8. c	13. f
4. b	9. g	14. a
5. b	10. c	15. b

EXERCISE 16.2 – OVERVIEW OF RADIOLOGY CODING

1. type of service; anatomic site; use of contrast material
2. technical
3. professional
4. global service
5. report (or results)

EXERCISE 16.3 – RADIOLOGY SECTION GUIDELINES

1. invasive
2. noninvasive
3. Surgical component: Introduction of catheter into the aorta (36200).
   Radiological component: Aortography radiological supervision and interpretation (75625).
4. intravascularly, intra-articularly, or intrathecally
5. False

EXERCISE 16.4 – DIAGNOSTIC RADIOLOGY (DIAGNOSTIC IMAGING)

1. 19102-RT, 77012   2. 70373   3. 75710-LT

> **Note:**
> - Do not assign code 75658-LT (instead of code 75710-LT) because there is no mention of a "retrograde" approach in the case. "Retrograde" means the contrast medium was injected "against the flow" of blood in the artery.
> - The surgeon would report the catheterization code (e.g., 36140-LT).

4. 72220   5. 76390

EXERCISE 16.5 – DIAGNOSTIC UTRASOUND

1. 76700
2. 76801
3. 76818
4. 76705
5. 76514
6. 47000, 77002, 36000
7. 61751, 77011
8. 20982-LT, 77022
9. 19102-LT, 77031
10. 77056

EXERCISE 16.6 – RADIATION ONCOLOGY

1. 77321
2. 77610
3. 77280
4. 77401

Note:

- Report code 77409 once because the description includes "two separate treatment areas."
- Do not report code 77427 (Radiation treatment management, five treatments) because although multiple areas received treatment, the delivery of radiation treatment in this case describes just one treatment. If the patient in this case underwent radiation treatment delivery on five separate occasions and the radiation oncologist documented radiation treatment management services, code 77427 would be reported in addition to code 77409.

5. 77789

EXERCISE 16.7 – NUCLEAR MEDICINE

1. 79101
2. 78195
3. 79403
4. 78587

Note:

- Anterior, posterior, and lateral views are considered multiple views.
- Do not report code 78588 (Pulmonary perfusion imaging, particulate, with ventilation imaging, aerosol, one or multiple projections). This case did not include documentation of "pulmonary perfusion imaging, particulate."

5. 78428

REVIEW

Multiple Choice

1. a
2. d
3. c
4. a
5. c
6. a
7. c
8. d
9. b
10. b
11. d
12. d
13. b
14. a
15. b
16. c
17. c
18. d
19. a
20. a

Coding Practice

21. 74000

> **Note:**
>
> *AP is the abbreviation for anteroposterior.*

22. 74270	27. 71100	31. 74410, 50394
23. 74290	28. 70250	32. 70240
24. 74245	29. 73120-LT	33. 72040
25. 74250	30. 71010	34. 73080-LT
26. 71020		

> **Note:**
>
> *A complete elbow x-ray includes a minimum of three views.*

35. 73562-50 (or 73562, 73562)

> **Note:**
>
> *Modifier -50 is approved for use with code 73562. However, it is also acceptable to report code 73562 two times on a claim.*

36. 73100-LT	39. 70120	42. 77402
37. 74010	40. 78205	43. 76870
38. 78635	41. 76805	44. 70491

> **Note:**
>
> *CT is the abbreviation for computed tomography.*

45. 72131	46. 73030	47. 78811

> **Note:**
>
> *PET is the abbreviation for positron emission tomography.*

48. 73610-LT	49. 75557

> **Note:**
>
> *MRI is the abbreviation for magnetic resonance imaging.*

50. 78306

Chapter 17
CPT Pathology and Laboratory

EXERCISE 17.1 – OVERVIEW OF PATHOLOGY AND LABORATORY SECTION

1. professional
2. methods
3. chargemaster
4. specimen
5. phlebotomy

6. 36415
7. 36400–36410
8. -26
9. -90

10. Clinical Laboratory Improvement Act of 1988 (CLIA)

EXERCISE 17.2 – PATHOLOGY AND LABORATORY SECTION GUIDELINES

1. specimen
2. twice

> **Note:**
>
> When multiple specimens are received for pathological examination, each specimen is considered a single unit of service and each is reported with a separate code. Thus, code 88302 is reported twice.

3. date of service
4. unlisted service or procedure; special report
5. -91; -51

EXERCISE 17.3 – PATHOLOGY AND LABORATORY SUBSECTIONS

1. 81000
2. 36415, 80162
3. 80051
4. 88331, 88331, 88332, 88305, 88305-59

> **Note:**
>
> • The frozen section of the first specimen is reported with code 88331.
> • The first frozen section on the second specimen is reported with code 88331, and the second frozen section for this specimen is reported with code 88332.
> • Code 88305 is reported twice to classify the two separately identified basal cell carcinomas for surgical pathology (definitive examination).

5. 81025   6. 36600, 82800   7. 82310, 82374, 82435, 82565, 84295, 84520

Note:

Do not report code 80048 (Basic metabolic panel) because potassium and glucose levels were not performed. A code for each laboratory test performed is reported separately: calcium (82310), carbon dioxide (82374), chloride (82435), creatinine (82565), sodium (84295), and urea nitrogen (BUN) (84520).

8. 88331, 88309   10. 36416, 82948   11. 88331, 88305
9. 85730

Note:

- The frozen section of this specimen is reported with code 88331.
- Surgical pathology evaluation of the breast biopsy is reported with code 88305.

12. 80061, 82947

Note:

- Code 80061 is reported for the lipid panel.
- Code 82947 is reported for the quantitative glucose test.

13. 80050

Note:

Code 80050 includes a hemogram. Therefore, a separate code is not reported for the hemogram.

14. 82374, 82435, 82565, 82947, 84132, 84295, 84520

Note:

- Do not report code 80053 (Comprehensive Metabolic Panel) because albumin, bilirubin (total), calcium, phosphatase (alkaline), protein (total), and transferase (alanine and aspartate amino) tests were not performed.
- Instead, each test is reported separately: carbon dioxide (82374), chloride (82435), creatinine (82565), glucose (82947), potassium (84132), sodium (84295), and urea nitrogen (BUN) (84520).

15. 86021   16. 87172   17. 88304

Note:

Although surgical pathology evaluation of appendix tissue is also included below code 88302, that code is for an incidental appendectomy (e.g., appendix removed incidentally during another procedure). For this case, the appendix was abnormal (due to acute appendicitis), which means that code 88304 is reported.

18. 87181   19. 89230

20. 88331, 88332, 88331-59, 88332-59, 88332-59, 88307, 88307-59, 88309

> **Note:**
> - The frozen section of two blocks from the right specimen are reported with codes 88331 and 88332.
> - The frozen section of three blocks from the left specimen are reported with codes 88331-59, 88332-59, and 88332-59.
> - Surgical pathology evaluation of right and left obturator lymph node resections are reported with codes 88307 and 88307-59.
> - Surgical pathology evaluation of prostate tissue (as the result of radical prostatectomy) is reported with code 88309.

REVIEW

Multiple Choice

1. a	7. c	13. b
2. b	8. b	14. c
3. c	9. b	15. d
4. c	10. b	16. c
5. d	11. a	17. d
6. a	12. a	

> **Note:**
> ABO, Rh, and MN blood typing are just 3 of 27 blood typing systems used to describe the absence or presence of antigens. (Many are named after the patients in whom they were initially encountered.)
> - ABO testing results in the determination of four principal blood group types: A, B, AB, and O.
> - Blood tested for the presence or absence of a Rhesis (Rh) blood protein results in Rh positive (Rh+) or Rh negative (Rh-) status.
> - The MN system tests for blood types M, N, or MN, which is useful in maternity and paternity testing.

18. d   19. d   20. a

Coding Practice

21. 80055

> **Note:**
> - The combination of these eight blood laboratory testing constitutes an obstetric panel. Assigning a separate code to each test is incorrect.
> - Rh(D) is the terminology used to identify a group of antigens on the surface of red blood cells.
> - ABO is the medical terminology used to classify blood types; A, B, AB, and O.
> - CBC is the abbreviation for complete blood count.
> - WBC is the abbreviation for white blood count.

22. 80069, 85027

Note:

- The ten tests—albumin, carbon dioxide, calcium, sodium, glucose, chloride, creatinine, urea nitrogen, potassium, and phosphorus inorganic—constitute a renal function panel.
- Because a CBC is not a part of a renal function panel, a separate code (85027) is assigned.

23. 81001   24. 89260, 89320

Note:

Code 89260 is reported for the sperm isolation procedure, and code 89320 is performed for semen analysis.

25. 80418

Note:

- These seven tests are done for suppression testing, and they are coded as a pituitary evaluation panel code.
- ACTH is the abbreviation for adrenocorticotropic hormone.
- HGH is the abbreviation for human growth hormone.
- TSH is the abbreviation for thyroid-stimulating hormone.
- LH is the abbreviation for luteinizing hormone.
- FSH is the abbreviation for follicle-stimulating hormone.

26. 87265   27. 87339

Note:

- H. pylori is the abbreviation for Helicobacter pylori.
- Code 87338 is assigned for H. pylori testing on stool or feces.

28. 85014   30. 88331   31. 87220
29. 82810

Note:

KOH is the abbreviation used to identify the method of using potassium hydroxide prep.

32. 84443, 84479   33. 80100   34. 86038

Note:

- ANA is the abbreviation for antinuclear antibodies.
- SLE is the abbreviation for systemic lupus erythematosus.

35. 88309

> **Note:**
> - The gross and microscopic exam of radically resected prostate tissue is coded to level VI under the Surgical Pathology subsection.
> - TURP is the abbreviation for transurethral resection of the prostate.

36. 86771   38. 86631   39. 88305
37. 84478

> **Note:**
> *The gross and microscopic exam of this type of tissue is classified as level IV below the Surgical Pathology subsection.*

40. 86485   41. 86901   42. 84153

> **Note:**
> *PSA is the abbreviation for prostate-specific antigen.*

43. 86359   44. 88304

> **Note:**
> *The examination of this type of tissue is classified as level III below the Surgical Pathology subsection.*

45. 86200

> **Note:**
> *CCP is the abbreviation for cyclic citrullinated peptide.*

46. 88029   48. 89050   49. 88230-5C
47. 88142

> **Note:**
> - Freidreich ataxia is a non-neoplastic disorder.
> - Modifier -5C is added to the code to identify the disorder (Freidreich ataxia in this case) that is being investigated via tissue analysis. Genetic testing modifiers are located in Appendix I of the CPT coding manual. They identify CPT codes that are reported for procedures performed for genetic testing purposes.

50. 88037

Chapter 18
CPT Medicine

EXERCISE 18.1 – INTRODUCTION AND OVERVIEW OF MEDICINE SECTION

1. noninvasive
2. minimally invasive
3. can
4. diagnostic and therapeutic
5. procedure-oriented

EXERCISE 18.2 – MEDICINE SECTION GUIDELINES

1. notes
2. separate
3. plus
4. separate procedure
5. HCPCS level II

EXERCISE 18.3 – MEDICINE SUBSECTIONS

1. 90473
2. 90822

> **Note:**
>
> Code 90822 includes individual psychotherapy (to modify the patient's obsessive-compulsive behavior) with medical evaluation and management services (performed to check the lithium blood levels).

3. 92980, 92981

> **Note:**
>
> Do not report codes 92982–92984 for coronary angioplasty or codes 92995–92996 for atherectomy. When performed in the same artery as the stent procedure, these procedures are included in the stent procedure codes (92980–92981).

4. 90954

> **Note:**
>
> Code is reported for each day when less than a full month (e.g., 30 days) of ESRD services are provided to a patient between age 2 and 11 years.

5. 96374

> **Note:**
>
> Neither of the IV flush procedures is coded and reported because an IV flush is integral to the infusion/injection service provided. HCPCS level II code J0696 is reported for each 250 mg dosage.

REVIEW

Multiple Choice

1. b	8. c	15. a
2. d	9. d	16. b
3. d	10. a	17. b
4. a	11. d	18. a
5. c	12. d	19. b
6. a	13. d	20. b
7. b	14. c	

Coding Practice

21. 92341	24. 91030	27. 94667
22. 96120	25. 93875	28. 93797
23. 92002	26. 92579	

Note:

There is no documentation that an ECG was performed during the procedure. Therefore, assign code 93797.

29. 90911

Note:

EMG is the abbreviation for electromyography.

30. 93288　　31. 93303

Note:

A ventricular septal defect (VSD) is a congenital heart condition.

32. 98941　　34. 97535, 97535　35. 95813
33. 90636, 90471

Note:

EEG is the abbreviation for electroencephalogram.

36. 91132　　37. 92516　　38. 90718, 90471

Note:

When assigning codes for the administration of immunizations or globulins, assign codes for administration of the injection and for the product being administered.

39. 90816   40. 93000   41. 92982, 92984

> **Note:**
>
> The procedure described in this note is a percutaneous transluminal coronary angioplasty (PTCA). Two vessels were treated, requiring assignment of codes 92982 and 92984. CPT code 92984 is an add-on code; therefore, do not add modifier -51.

42. 93015

> **Note:**
>
> ECG is the abbreviation for electrocardiogram.

43. 91105   44. 99503   45. 97001

> **Note:**
>
> CVA is the abbreviation for cerebrovascular accident.

46. 95125   47. 96920   48. 90375, 90772

> **Note:**
>
> IM is the abbreviation for intramuscular.

49. 90921   50. 96413, 96415

> **Note:**
>
> IV is the abbreviation for intravenous.

Chapter 19
Insurance and Reimbursement

EXERCISE 19.1 – THIRD-PARTY PAYERS

1. Medicare administrative contractors (MAC)
2. Centers for Medicare & Medicaid Services (CMS)
3. CMS-1500; UB-92 or CMS-1450 (UB-04 in 2007)
4. clearinghouse
5. hold harmless clause
6. CHAMPVA
7. Medicaid
8. Medicare
9. managed care
10. fee-for-service

EXERCISE 19.2 – HEALTH CARE REIMBURSEMENT SYSTEMS

1. $1,200 ($1,500 × 80%); $300 ($1,500 × 20%).
2. $4,480 ([$1,400 × 4] × 80% = $4,480); $4,500, which is the DRG prospective payment amount
3. chargemaster review
4. Tax Equity and Fiscal Responsibility Act of 1983 (TEFRA)
5. ambulatory payment classifications (APCs)
6. a
7. a
8. b
9. b
10. a

EXERCISE 19.3 – IMPACT OF HIPAA ON REIMBURSEMENT

1. a
2. b
3. b
4. a
5. a
6. national health plan identifier (PlanID)
7. national standard employer identifier number (EIN)
8. national provider identifier (NPI)
9. electronic data interchange (EDI)
10. security

REVIEW

Multiple Choice

1. c	8. b	15. b
2. a	9. a	16. b
3. b	10. d	17. b
4. d	11. d	18. d
5. c	12. c	19. c
6. b	13. b	20. c
7. b	14. c	

Chapter Exams and Answer Keys to Chapter Exams

Chapter 1
Overview of Coding

1. An at-home coding specialist enters manifestation codes into the computer. Which type of HIPAA code set is being used?
   a. ASP
   b. CPT
   c. large
   d. SNOMED CT

2. A facility enters into a contract with a billing service to convert health information and claims from a nonstandard to a standard format. The billing service is considered a:
   a. health care clearinghouse.
   b. health care plan.
   c. third-party administrator.
   d. third-party payer.

3. A claims examiner reviews a patient's chart to locate documentation of a diagnosis to justify treatment provided. What is the examiner trying to establish?
   a. medical coding
   b. medical necessity
   c. medical nomenclature
   d. medical record

4. Which coding system is currently used in the United States?
   a. DSM-III
   b. ICD-O-3
   c. ICD-10
   d. ICDA

5. The medical record is considered a _____ for a patient encounter.
   a. business record
   b. financial record
   c. medical nomenclature
   d. registration report

6. Secondary purposes of the medical record:
   a. do not relate directly to patient care.
   b. have as an option, medicolegal purposes.
   c. include the planning of individual patient care.
   d. usually do not require accurate documentation.

7. Which of the following statements about a student internship is true?
   a. Because students are not considered employees, they do not have to adhere to a dress code.
   b. Breach of confidentiality can result in termination from the internship site.
   c. Sometimes students receive monetary compensation for their work.
   d. Students must submit a professional resume to the facility supervisor.

8. A student is preparing to sit for a credentialing exam offered through the American Health Information Management Association. Which is the student pursuing?
   a. Certified Coding Specialist
   b. Certified Professional Coder
   c. Electronic Claims Professional
   d. Registered Medical Assistant

9. Students join their professional organizations:
   a. after they graduate.
   b. only if they are sponsored by a member.
   c. to receive all of the benefits provided to active members.
   d. usually for a reduced fee.

10. A health care professional would like to network with other professionals via the Internet. Which would be most helpful for this purpose?
    a. ASP
    b. hyperlink
    c. listerv
    d. WAN

11. Which nomenclature is in use today?
    a. CMIT
    b. SNDO
    c. SNOMED CT
    d. SNOP

12. Which coding system would a physician's office most likely use?
    a. CDT
    b. CPT
    c. DSM
    d. NDC

13. Susan just attended a lecture on new procedures and techniques used in cardiac care, and she received continuing education (CE) credits for her participation. How will CE credits professionally benefit Susan?
    a. Susan can apply the CE credits towards maintenance of her professional credential.
    b. Susan can use CE credits to earn a degree in the coding profession.
    c. Susan can use CE credits to earn a professional credential.
    d. Susan's CE credits are required to maintain her professional degree.

14. A coding specialist is more likely to be credentialed by:
    a. AHIMA.
    b. AMT.
    c. MAB.
    d. NEBA.

15. Which problem-oriented record SOAP note is documented for the statement "Patient's diagnosis is acute bronchitis"?
    a. subjective
    b. objective
    c. assessment
    d. plan

16. Which problem-oriented record SOAP note is documented for the statement "Chest x-ray reveals areas of lung consolidation"?
    a. subjective
    b. objective
    c. assessment
    d. plan

17. Which problem-oriented record SOAP note is documented for the statement "Patient complains of headache"?
    a. subjective
    b. objective
    c. assessment
    d. plan

18. Which problem-oriented record SOAP note is documented for the statement "Patient is scheduled for brain scan on Tuesday?"
    a. subjective
    b. objective
    c. assessment
    d. plan

19. The physician documents "acute and chronic asthma" on the patient's record. Which coding system is used to assign codes for claims submission?
    a. CPT
    b. HCPCS level I
    c. HCPCS level II
    d. ICD-9-CM

20. Which credentialing exam is offered by the American Academy of Professional Coders?
    a. CCA
    b. CCS
    c. CMRS
    d. CPC

Chapter 2
Introduction to ICD-9-CM Coding

1. The Medicare Prescription Drug, Improvement, and Modernization Act (MMA) requires ICD-9-CM codes to be updated:
   a. after a 90-day grace period so computer systems can be updated.
   b. annually; and updated codes must be implemented immediately.
   c. as the cooperating parties for the ICD-9-CM make monthly changes.
   d. each April 1 and October 1; and they must be implemented immediately.

2. Which mandated the reporting of ICD-9-CM diagnosis codes on Medicare claims?
   a. cooperating parties for the ICD-9-CM
   b. Medicare Catastrophic Coverage Act of 1988
   c. Medicare Prescription Drug, Improvement, and Modernization Act
   d. third-party payers, including commercial insurance companies

3. Which automates the coding process using computerized or Web-based software?
   a. encoder
   b. grouper
   c. maximizer
   d. optimizer

4. Which supplementary classification would be referenced to code a homicide attempt?
   a. Contact with health services
   b. External cause of injury
   c. Factors influencing health status
   d. Morphology of neoplasms

5. Subterms, which are indented two spaces below main terms, are also called _____ modifiers.
   a. essential
   b. necessary
   c. nonessential
   d. secondary

6. To initially locate an E code, go to the:
   a. Alphabetic Index to External Causes of Injury and Poisoning.
   b. Index of Diseases.
   c. Supplemental Classification of Factors Influencing Health Status and Contact with Health Services.
   d. Table of Drugs and Chemicals.

7. ICD-9-CM Volume 3 includes a(n):
   a. alphabetical index of all outpatient procedures and services.
   b. alphanumeric anatomic listing of inpatient procedures and services.
   c. tabular list of 17 chapters.
   d. Tabular List of Procedures and Index to Procedures.

8. The ICD-9-CM Tabular List of Procedures chapters are arranged:
   a. according to anatomic site.
   b. alphabetically.
   c. by service or procedure.
   d. numerically.

9. The cooperating parties for the ICD-9-CM approve guidelines that have been prepared for coding and reporting using the ICD-9-CM and consist of which organizations?
   a. AHA, AHIMA, CMS, and NCHS
   b. APA, AHIMA, DHHS, and AHA
   c. MMA, CMS, APA, and NCHS
   d. WHO, DHHS, AHIMA, CMS, and NCHS

10. The guidelines prepared by the cooperating parties for the ICD-9-CM:
    a. are required by the Medicare Prescription Drug, Improvement, and Modernization Act (MMA).
    b. contain rules for the Tabular List of Diseases only.

    c. had been developed to override the official conventions in ICD-9-CM.

    d. include coding and sequencing instructions for ICD-9-CM.

11. ICD-9-CM Index to Diseases subterms are indented _____ spaces with respect to main terms.

    a. two   c. five

    b. four   d. six

12. Within the ICD-9-CM Tabular List of Diseases, which contain groups of three-digit categories?

    a. categories   c. subcategories

    b. sections   d. subclassifications

13. "Persons with health hazards related to communicable diseases" is an example of a(n):

    a. chapter in the ICD-9-CM Tabular List of Diseases.

    b. chapter in the ICD-9-CM Tabular List of Procedures.

    c. ICD-9-CM grouping of E codes.

    d. ICD-9-CM grouping of V codes.

14. "Place of occurrence" is an example of a:

    a. chapter in the ICD-9-CM Tabular List of Diseases.

    b. chapter in the ICD-9-CM Tabular List of Procedures.

    c. grouping of ICD-9-CM E codes.

    d. grouping of ICD-9-CM V codes.

15. To properly assign a code from the ICD-9-CM neoplasm table when a diagnosis is documented as "neoplasm of the pyloric antrum," the coder should:

    a. assign a code from the Unspecified column.

    b. contact the state cancer registry for clarification.

    c. refer to the morphology entry in the Index to Diseases.

    d. review the pathology report to determine the type of neoplasm.

16. The ICD-9-CM Table of Drugs and Chemicals contains a main entry for "Drug," which:

    a. can be referenced when the AHFS list number has not been provided.

    b. contains a list of drugs that are not listed elsewhere in the Table of Drugs and Chemicals.

    c. directs the coder to Appendix C of the ICD-9-CM coding manual.

    d. lists drugs according to the American Hospital Formulary Services (AHFS) list number.

17. The Tabular List of Diseases should be referenced:

    a. for verification of E codes and V codes only.

    b. if the phrase *omit code* is included in the index.

    c. to verify codes selected and to review instructions.

    d. when a procedure code is listed as unspecified.

18. Which connecting term(s) immediately follow the main term to which they refer in the ICD-9-CM Index to Procedures?

    a. *by*   c. *to*

    b. *for*   d. *with and without*

19. The phrase *omit code* located after a main term or subterm in the ICD-9-CM Index to Procedures indicates that the operative approach is:

    a. considered an integral part of the procedure, and it is coded.

    b. considered an integral part of the procedure, and it is not coded.

    c. not considered an integral part of the procedure, and it is coded.

    d. not considered an integral part of the procedure, and it is not coded.

20. After locating a code in the ICD-9-CM Index to Procedures, the coder's next step is to:

    a. link the procedure code to a diagnosis code.

    b. locate that code in the Tabular List of Procedures to review instructions and verify the code.

    c. locate the main term in the Index to Procedures.

    d. review the code description in the Tabular List of Procedures to determine if the "omit code" instruction applies.

Chapter 3
ICD-9-CM Coding Conventions

1. ICD-9-CM Index to Diseases subterms are indented _____ spaces below main terms.
   a. two
   b. four
   c. five
   d. six

2. Where would the abbreviation NEC (not elsewhere classifiable) be found in ICD-9-CM?
   a. Index to Diseases and Index to Procedures
   b. Index to Diseases and Tabular List of Diseases
   c. Index to Procedures and Tabular List of Procedures
   d. Tabular List of Diseases and Tabular List of Procedures

3. Where would the abbreviation NOS (not otherwise specified) be found in ICD-9-CM?
   a. Index to Diseases and Index to Procedures
   b. Tabular List of Diseases and Index to Diseases
   c. Tabular List of Diseases and Tabular List of Procedures
   d. Tabular List of Procedures and Index to Procedures

4. Which are used in the ICD-9-CM Index to Diseases to identify manifestation codes?
   a. colons
   b. parentheses
   c. slanted brackets
   d. square brackets

5. The ICD-9-CM _____ contains "includes" notes.
   a. Index to Diseases
   b. Index to Procedures
   c. Table of Drugs and Chemicals
   d. Tabular List of Diseases and Tabular List of Procedures

6. The appearance of an "excludes" note beneath an ICD-9-CM code indicates that:
   a. codes for excluded conditions are always to be reported with the code from which the condition is excluded.
   b. codes for excluded conditions are never to be reported with the code from which the condition is excluded.
   c. codes for excluded conditions may or may not be reported with the code from which the condition is excluded.
   d. the coder must assign an unspecified code number to the condition.

7. Inclusion terms are:
   a. antonyms of the code title or for "unspecified" codes, are a list of conditions assigned to that code.
   b. exhaustive; so if the correct term is not listed below the code, that code cannot be assigned.
   c. listed below certain four- and five-digit ICD-9-CM codes in the Index to Diseases and the Index to Procedures.
   d. listed below certain four- and five-digit ICD-9-CM codes in the Tabular List of Diseases and the Tabular List of Procedures.

8. An ICD-9-CM "other specified" code:
   a. generally contains a fourth digit of 9 and/or a fifth digit of 0.
   b. is sufficient to assign a more specific code.
   c. requires the reporting of multiple codes for a case.
   d. usually contains a fourth and/or fifth digit of 8 and/or 9.

9. The relationship between etiology and manifestation codes results in the:
   a. correct sequencing of the manifestation code first, followed by the etiology code.
   b. etiology code being printed in slanted brackets in the Index to Diseases.
   c. etiology code being reported first, followed by the manifestation code.
   d. manifestation code defining the underlying condition or disease.

10. The "see also" instruction in ICD-9-CM:
    a. appears in the Tabular List of Diseases and is an optional guideline.
    b. does not have to be followed if the original main term provides the correct code.
    c. is considered a mandatory optional guideline in the Index to Diseases.
    d. must be followed for disease and procedure codes to be assigned properly.

11. Which must be included in the diagnostic statement to classify a condition or procedure?
    a. inclusion terms
    b. modifier included after the colon
    c. nonessential modifiers enclosed in parentheses
    d. synonyms enclosed in square brackets

12. A patient is diagnosed with phlyctenulosis due to tuberculosis. Codes 017.3 and [370.31] are located in the Index to Diseases. Upon verification in the Tabular List of Diseases, report code(s):
    a. 017.3 with an appropriate fifth digit only.
    b. 017.3 with an appropriate fifth digit and 370.31 in that order.
    c. 370.31 only.
    d. 370.31 and 017.3 with an appropriate fifth digit in that order.

13. The description for code 460 in the Tabular List of Diseases is "acute nasopharyngitis [common cold]." How is this code description interpreted?
    a. Acute nasopharyngitis and common cold are synonymous.
    b. acute nasopharyngitis due to common cold
    c. acute nasopharyngitis with common cold
    d. common cold due to acute nasopharyngitis

14. Which contain nonessential modifiers that may be present or absent in the provider's diagnostic statement?
    a. parentheses   c. square brackets
    b. slanted brackets   d. tables

15. ICD-9-CM coding conventions are:
    a. based on official coding guidelines.
    b. chapter-specific rules used to code diseases and procedures.
    c. incorporated into ICD-9-CM as instructional notes.
    d. used only in the Tabular List of Diseases.

16. The concept "trust the index" means that:
    a. if a term has been used to correctly locate a code in the Index to Diseases but that term is not described in the Tabular List of Diseases code entry, trust that the index directed you to the correct code.
    b. all terms that apply to a particular code will be listed in the tabular list code description; thus, if there is no inclusion term for that condition, the code cannot be assigned.
    c. inclusion terms located in the Index to Diseases are not meant to be exhaustive, and additional terms found in the Tabular List of Diseases may also be associated with a code.
    d. if a term has been used to correctly locate a code in the Index to Diseases and the code listed in the index contains a fifth digit, it is not necessary to verify the code in the Tabular List of Diseases.

17. The concept of "moving up the ladder" of codes in the tabular list means:
    a. assigning the proper codes to ensure that maximum reimbursement is obtained for the facility.
    b. ensuring that a fifth digit is always assigned when one is available for that code in the Tabular List of Diseases.

c. reviewing the record or asking the physician for clarification of documentation to determine whether a more specific code can be assigned.

d. sequencing codes so the first-listed code reflects the reason for the encounter and secondary codes list additional diagnoses, complications, and comorbidities.

18. Which instruction is optional when a secondary condition is not documented?
    a. code first underlying condition
    b. code, if applicable, any causal condition first
    c. in diseases classified elsewhere
    d. use additional code

19. Which is listed alphabetically according to main term in the Index to Diseases?
    a. External Causes of Injury and Poisoning
    b. Index to Procedures
    c. Neoplasm Table
    d. Table of Drugs and Chemicals

20. Boxed notes provide information or instruction in the Index to Diseases and Index to Procedures. Which functions of boxed notes are associated with the Index to Diseases but *not* with the Index to Procedures? Boxed notes:
    a. identify manifestation codes.
    b. include nonessential modifiers.
    c. list fifth-digit subclassifications for those categories that use the same fifth digits.
    d. provide coding instruction.

Chapter 4
ICD-9-CM Coding Guidelines

1. Which procedure requires the assignment of an ICD-9-CM code for the surgical approach?
   a. Exploratory laparotomy to remove mass, but surgery is halted.
   b. Neurosurgeon performed a craniotomy and removed a brain lesion.
   c. Surgeon made a laparotomy incision and performed a laparoscopic appendectomy.
   d. Surgeon made a skin incision and performed a vein stripping procedure.

2. A symptomatic HIV-positive patient is admitted to the hospital following a motor vehicle accident. The patient is diagnosed as having an open fracture of the femoral shaft and undergoes open reduction with internal fixation. The patient receives HIV antiviral medication while in the hospital.
   a. 042
   b. 042, 821.11
   c. 821.11
   d. 821.11, 042

3. A patient with chronic choroiditis presents with complaints of decreased vision. The patient is diagnosed with cataract due to choroiditis.
   a. 363.20
   b. 366.32
   c. 363.20, 366.32
   d. 366.32, 363.20

4. A patient was admitted after an accidental industrial explosion occurred at his workplace, resulting in a fire. The patient sustained second-degree burns of the right ear, second- and third-degree burns of the shoulder, and first- and second-degree burns of the hand; Twenty percent of the body sustained burns, with 10% third-degree burns, 20% second-degree burns, and 5% first-degree burns.
   a. 941.21, 943.25, 943.35, 944.10, 944.20, 948.21, E891.3
   b. 941.21, 943.35, 944.20, 948.21, E891.3
   c. 943.35, 941.21, 944.20, 948.21, E891.3
   d. 943.35, 943.25, 944.20, 941.21, 943.13, 948.21, E891.3

5. A patient had an encounter with his family doctor to receive a preemployment physical examination and was diagnosed with an external ear infection.
   a. 380.10
   b. 380.10, V70.5
   c. V70.5
   d. V70.5, 380.10

6. A woman was admitted to the hospital in labor, and she delivered. The final diagnoses included uterine pregnancy, delivery of oversized infant with low forceps and episiotomy; and postdelivery hematoma of episiotomy.
   a. 653.51, 674.31, V27.0, 72.1
   b. 653.51, 674.32, V27.0, 72.1
   c. 653.51, 674.32, V27.0, 72.9
   d. 674.32, 653.51, V27.0, 72.1

7. A patient recently underwent a mastectomy for treatment of an upper/inner quadrant adenocarcinoma of the breast. Today the patient has an outpatient encounter for radiation therapy.
   a. 174.2
   b. 174.2, V58.0
   c. V58.0
   d. V58.0, 174.2

8. A patient presents with complaint of pain and stiffness in the left ankle. The diagnosis is documented as traumatic arthritis of the ankle.
   a. 716.17, 908.9
   b. 716.17, 959.7
   c. 908.9, 716.17
   d. 959.7, 716.17

9. A patient is admitted with complaints of chest pain and shortness of breath. During the exam, the patient revealed that he had recently come into contact with a white powdery substance in his duties as a postal employee and that a coworker had contracted anthrax. After examination, the physician diagnosed the patient with pneumonia due to pulmonary anthrax.
   a. 022.1, 484.5, E915
   b. 022.1, 484.5, E979.6
   c. 484.5, 022.1, E915
   d. 484.5, 022.1, E979.6

10. Which of the following is classified by assigning an adverse effect code from the ICD-9-CM Table of Drugs and Chemicals?
   a. A patient was admitted in a comatose state. The patient's brother said that an empty bottle of Tylenol with Codeine, which had just been filled that morning, was found on the table beside the patient. The patient had threatened to hurt herself the day before.
   b. A patient was prescribed Percocet for back pain due to a muscle injury and was admitted after a motor vehicle accident. The patient claimed that he wasn't getting enough relief from the pain, so he took an "extra dose" that morning and must have fallen asleep at the wheel.
   c. A patient who takes prescribed doses of diclofenac for arthritis frequently takes aspirin for headaches. She is admitted to the hospital with gastrointestinal bleeding.
   d. A patient with back pain due to a displaced disk was prescribed Darvocet. While taking prescribed doses, the patient experienced extreme fatigue and bradycardia.

11. A patient is diagnosed as having renal and heart disease due to hypertension.
   a. 402.90, 403.90
   b. 404.90
   c. 404.90, 401.9
   d. 404.90, 402.90, 403.90

12. A pregnant woman underwent outpatient termination of a pregnancy. The diagnosis was elective abortion due to maternal rubella. Aspiration curettage was performed.
   a. 635.92, 647.5, 69.51
   b. 635.92, 655.30, 69.51
   c. 635.92, 655.33, 69.52
   d. 655.33, 635.90, 69.51

13. A patient had an encounter for the fitting and adjustment of his artificial arm.
   a. 682.3, V52.0
   b. V52.0
   c. V52.0, 682.3
   d. V52.0, 887.4

14. The patient is a toddler who was traveling, unrestrained, in a motor vehicle driven by the patient's mother. A bee flew through the open window of the vehicle and stung the driver, causing her to veer off the road and hit a tree. The patient sustained multiple contusions and abrasions and a facial laceration. Which is the proper sequencing of E code(s) for this encounter?
   a. E905.3, E816.1
   b. E816.1, E905.3
   c. E816.1, E967.2
   d. E967.2, E816.1

15. A 5-hour-old infant, premature at 30 weeks, spontaneous birth, is transferred to the hospital's neonatal intensive care unit. Final diagnoses include male newborn; suspected respiratory disease due to prematurity.
   a. 765.10, 769
   b. 765.10, V71.89
   c. V30.00, 765.10
   d. V30.00, 765.25, 769

16. Which procedure requires the assignment of an ICD-9-CM screening code?
   a. A seemingly well 52-year-old woman has an encounter for an occult blood test.
   b. A woman has an encounter for a routine postpartum examination.
   c. During an encounter, a patient states that he had poliomyelitis when he was young.
   d. Patient is admitted for observation for suspected tuberculosis.

17. A patient was admitted for the repair of a hiatal hernia by abdominal approach. The patient, who suffers from chronic paranoid schizophrenia, became agitated and, after consultation, received treatment for acute exacerbation of the condition.
   a. 553.3, 295.30, 53.7
   b. 553.3, 295.34, 53.7
   c. 553.3, 53.7
   d. 750.6, 295.34, 53.7

18. A patient is admitted for breathing treatments due to acute exacerbation of chronic obstructive pulmonary disease (COPD) with asthma.
    a. 493.22
    b. 493.82
    c. 493.92, 496
    d. 496, 493.92

19. The patient was admitted for open biopsy of the frontal nasal sinus. Open biopsy was performed, and frozen section results from pathology were positive for cancer. The patient underwent an excision of the frontal sinus lesion during the same operative episode.
    a. 22.12, 22.42
    b. 22.12
    c. 22.42
    d. 22.42, 22.12

20. The patient fell while climbing a tree and sustained a concussion, along with numerous contusions of the face, arms, and legs. The patient also sustained a laceration on the left leg.
    a. 850.9, 891.0, E884.9
    b. 850.9, 891.0, 923.9, 920, E884.9
    c. 850.9, 891.0, 923.9, 924.5, 920, E884.9
    d. 923.9, 920, 850.9, 891.0, E884.9

Chapter 5
ICD-9-CM Hospital Inpatient Coding

1. A patient is admitted as a hospital inpatient for open reduction of fractured femur, sustained during a fall at home. The patient was also treated for congestive heart failure during the inpatient stay.
   a. 428.0, 79.25, E888.9, E849.0
   b. 428.0, 820.8, E888.9, E849.0, 79.25
   c. 820.8, 428.0, E888.9, E849.0
   d. 820.8, 428.0, E888.9, E849.0, 79.25

2. A patient underwent total left knee replacement surgery for severe osteoarthritis, left knee, as a hospital inpatient. Her inpatient stay was extended when a postoperative wound infection developed, which cultured as methicillin-resistant Staphylococcus aureus. The patient received successful intravenous antibiotic therapy for treatment of the infection and was discharged.
   a. 041.11, 715.96, 998.59, V09.0, 81.54, 99.29
   b. 715.96, 041.11, 998.59, V09.0, 81.54, 99.29
   c. 715.96, 998.59, 041.11, V09.0, 81.54, 99.29
   d. 998.59, 041.11, 715.96, V09.0, 81.54, 99.29

3. A patient underwent below-knee amputation of the left leg as a hospital inpatient due to peripheral vascular disease secondary to type 2 diabetes mellitus.
   a. 250.70, 443.8, 84.15
   b. 443.81, 250.70, 84.15
   c. 250.70, 443.81, 84.15
   d. V49.75, 84.15, 84.3

4. A hospital inpatient underwent sigmoidectomy with creation of temporary colostomy due to obstruction, which was determined to be carcinoma of the colon. The patient received his first round of chemotherapy during his inpatient stay.
   a. 560.9, V58.11, 45.76, 46.11
   b. 751.2, V58.11, 45.76, 46.11
   c. 997.4, V58.11, 45.76, 46.11
   d. 159.0, V58.11, 45.76, 46.11

5. A patient is seen in the emergency department for high fever, chills, abdominal pain, and vomiting and is then admitted to the hospital with a diagnosis of septicemia due to pseudomonas with septic shock.
   a. 038.43
   b. 038.43, 785.52
   c. 038.43, 995.92, 785.52
   d. 995.92, 038.43, 785.52

6. The patient was admitted to the hospital for acute treatment of decubitus bedsores of both hips.
   a. 707.00
   b. 707.04
   c. 707.07
   d. 707.09

7. A patient suffering from weight loss and fatigue is diagnosed with pancreatic cancer and anemia due to impaired absorption. The patient is admitted to the hospital and undergoes radical pancreatectomy.
   a. 157.9, 280.9, 52.7
   b. 157.9, 285.9, 52.7
   c. 157.9, 783.21, 780.79, 285.9, 52.7
   d. 783.21, 780.79, 157.9, 285.9, 52.7

8. A patient with acute cholecystitis was admitted to the hospital and underwent cholecystectomy. Postoperatively, the patient developed adult respiratory distress syndrome (ARDS).
   a. 518.5, 575.0, 51.04
   b. 575.0, 518.5, 51.04
   c. 575.0, 518.5, 51.22
   d. 575.10, 518.5, 51.04

9. A patient was admitted to the hospital for gastric ulcer with hemorrhage and perforation, which resulted in acute anemia.
   a. 531.6, 285.1
   b. 531.6, 285.9
   c. 531.60, 285.1
   d. 531.9, 459.0, 285.9

10. A patient with HIV disease was admitted with a stab wound to the thoracic aorta, which resulted when the patient fell on a pitchfork that was hidden in hay. The wound was repaired with synthetic graft material.
    a. 042, 901.0, E920.4, 39.57
    b. 042, 901.0, E966, 39.57
    c. 879.8, 042, E920.4, 39.57
    d. 901.0, 042, E920.4, 39.57

11. A female patient is admitted with intrauterine pregnancy at term. Because of cephalopelvic disproportion, a cesarean section was performed, and a healthy male infant was delivered.
    a. 653.41, V27.0, 74.99
    b. 653.41, V27.0
    c. 660.11, 653.41, 74.99
    d. 660.11, 653.41, V27.0, 74.99

12. During the same inpatient admission, a full-term infant was born and subsequently developed an upper respiratory infection (URI) and physiologic jaundice.
    a. 465.9, 774.6
    b. 465.9, 774.6, V30.00
    c. V30.00, 465.9
    d. V30.00, 465.9, 774.6

13. A Parkinson patient is admitted to the hospital with a urinary tract infection due to Escherichia coli and dehydration. The patient received treatment for all of these conditions.
    a. 332.0, 599.0, 276.51, 041.4
    b. 599.0, 041.4, 276.51, 332.0
    c. 599.0, 041.4, 332.0
    d. 599.0, 276.51, 332.0

14. A patient is admitted to the hospital and undergoes resection of congenital hallux valgus. To stabilize the foot during healing, the patient is fitted for a below-knee cast.
    a. 727.1, 77.59
    b. 735.0, 77.59, 93.53
    c. 755.56, 77.59
    d. 755.66, 77.59, 93.53

15. A 17-hour-old infant weighing 1000 grams and premature at 30 weeks via spontaneous birth was transferred to Alfred State Medical Center's neonatal intensive care unit (NICU). Final diagnoses include female newborn and suspected respiratory disease due to prematurity.
    a. 765.14, 765.25, 769
    b. 765.14, 769
    c. 765.14, 765.25
    d. 765.14, V71.89

16. A patient is admitted with acute coronary insufficiency of the right coronary artery with hypertensive heart disease. Percutaneous transluminal coronary angioplasty (PTCA) with insertion of coronary stent is performed.
    a. 411.89, 402.90, 00.66, 36.06, 00.45, 00.40
    b. 411.89, 402.90, 36.01, 36.06, 00.45, 00.40
    c. 411.89, 402.90, 36.06, 00.45, 00.40
    d. 411.89, 402.90, 39.50, 36.06

17. A patient was brought to the hospital by ambulance and admitted for cerebrovascular accident (CVA) secondary to cerebral embolism with infarction.
    a. 434.11
    b. 436
    c. 436, 434.11, 437.9
    d. 437.9

18. A patient is admitted to the hospital and undergoes repair of cleft palate. The patient is a child who is severely mentally retarded and receives appropriate treatment for this condition during the hospitalization.
    a. 318.1, 749.00, 27.62
    b. 318.1, 749.00, 27.64
    c. 749.00, 27.64
    d. 749.00, 318.1, 27.62

19. A woman who receives treatment for depression is brought to the emergency department with complaints of acute pelvic pain and nausea, which began one hour prior to admission. She was taken to surgery and underwent left oophorectomy. The postoperative diagnosis was torsion of the ovary. The patient received medication for her depression and for Hashimoto thyroiditis during the hospitalization.
    a. 311, 620.5, 245.2, 65.39
    b. 620.5, 311, 245.2
    c. 620.5, 311, 245.2, 65.39
    d. 620.5, 65.39

20. An unconscious patient is admitted with cerebral anoxia due to previous overdose of sedatives (AHFS 28:24) as a suicide attempt. During this admission, the patient receives treatment for cerebral anoxia.
    a. 348.1, 909.0, E950.2
    b. 348.1, 909.0, E959
    c. 348.1, E950.2
    d. 799.0, 909.0, E959

Chapter 6
ICD-9-CM Outpatient and Physician Office Coding

1. Qualified diagnoses are a necessary part of a patient's hospital and office record; however, physician offices are required to report:
   a. qualified diagnoses for inpatients and outpatients.
   b. qualified diagnoses related to outpatient procedures.
   c. signs and symptoms in addition to qualified diagnoses.
   d. signs and symptoms instead of qualified diagnoses.

2. Brenda submitted a Medicare claim on which the first-listed diagnosis code was V57.3 (encounter for speech therapy) and the second-listed code was 784.3 (aphasia). The Medicare administrative contractor (MAC) denied the claim, stating that its policy was not to pay claims that report V codes first. Brenda contacted the MAC and explained that she knew this claim was submitted correctly and in accordance with CMS's *Diagnostic Coding and Reporting Guidelines for Outpatient Services: Hospital-Based and Physician Office*. The MAC's representative repeated the policy and would not process the claim to provide reimbursement to the physician. Brenda then contacted her regional CMS office for resolution and relayed the details of the incident. How would you summarize the way Brenda handled this situation?
   a. Brenda's actions were partially warranted, but she should never contact CMS.
   b. Brenda's actions were warranted; but before contacting CMS, she should have provided the MAC with information about the HIPAA provision that requires compliance with the ICD-9-CM official coding guidelines.
   c. Brenda's actions were completely unwarranted because the MAC can decide what claims to reimburse based on internal policies.
   d. Brenda's actions were completely warranted because she knew she had submitted a clean claim and the MAC should stay current regarding HIPAA regulations.

3. If an examination is for administrative purposes (e.g., preemployment physical) and it is not focused on any particular condition, which additional ICD-9-CM codes may be reported?
   a. chronic conditions
   b. chronic conditions and history of codes
   c. preexisting conditions and history of codes
   d. preexisting conditions, chronic conditions, and history of codes

4. Which V code category is reportable as a first-listed diagnosis?
   a. V09, infection with drug-resistant microorganisms
   b. V41, problems with special senses and other special functions
   c. V42, organ or tissue replaced by transplant
   d. V59, donors

5. Signs and symptoms should be coded when _____.
   a. a definitive diagnosis has been established by the physician.
   b. a qualified diagnosis has been confirmed by the physician.
   c. they are not routinely associated with the disease process that initiated the encounter.
   d. they are part of the disease process that initiated the encounter.

6. Etiology/manifestation coding may require the assignment of _____.
   a. a history code
   b. a late effect code
   c. an E code
   d. more than one code

159

7. A patient is treated for dysphagia, which is a late effect of the poliomyelitis he had several years ago. How would this be coded?
   a. Assign a code for dysphagia and a code for late effect of poliomyelitis.
   b. Code only the dysphagia.
   c. Report codes for poliomyelitis, dysphagia, and late effect of poliomyelitis, in that order.
   d. Report poliomyelitis as the first-listed code and dysphagia as an additional code.

8. Which describes the condition chiefly responsible for services provided during an outpatient visit?
   a. encounter
   b. first-listed diagnosis
   c. principal diagnosis
   d. qualified diagnosis

9. History codes (V10–V19) may be reported as secondary codes if the historical condition or family history has an impact on current care or influences treatment. Reporting history codes _____ reimbursement.
   a. always increases
   b. could increase
   c. decreases
   d. never impacts

10. A patient is seen in the physician's office with the complaint of a sore throat. The physician orders lab tests and documents "pharyngitis, rule out strep infection." The next day the lab results are interpreted by the physician, whose report lists "influenza with pharyngitis" as the diagnosis. Which condition(s) are reported on the outpatient claim?
    a. influenza
    b. influenza with pharyngitis
    c. pharyngitis with strep throat
    d. sore throat

11. Preadmission testing (PAT):
    a. can be performed only for outpatient surgery.
    b. could result in higher reimbursement to a health care facility.
    c. does not facilitate the patient's treatment.
    d. is performed only for inpatient admissions.

12. A patient with pelvic pain underwent outpatient laser laparoscopy for suspected ovarian cysts. During the procedure, no cysts were found; but endometriosis was discovered and documented as the postoperative diagnosis. Which is reported on the outpatient claim?
    a. endometriosis
    b. endometriosis and pelvic pain
    c. ovarian cysts
    d. pelvic pain

13. Which is reported when an outpatient diagnostic test is performed to confirm a suspected condition and the test rules out the condition?
    a. confirmed diagnosis
    b. qualified diagnosis
    c. screening code
    d. signs and symptoms

14. A patient presents with back pain and is referred for magnetic resonance imaging (MRI) to rule out a herniated disk. The interpreted MRI report confirms a herniated disk. However, the encounter was coded as back pain. Which would be an acceptable reason for this code assignment?
    a. The reason for the encounter is all that should be coded.
    b. The coder did not review the entire chart before assigning codes.
    c. The physician's interpretation of the test result is unclear, and the physician was unavailable for clarification.
    d. The report containing the interpretation of the MRI was not available at the time the claim was processed.

15. A patient is referred for an x-ray for suspected rib fracture. After reviewing the x-ray, the interpreting physician confirms the rib fracture and also discovers spots on a lung. How should this be coded?
    a. Only the fractured rib is coded because the spots on the lung are incidental.
    b. Only the spots on the lung are coded because they require immediate intervention.
    c. The fractured rib is coded and reported first, and the spots on the lung are coded and reported second because they are an incidental finding.
    d. The spots on the lung are coded and reported first because they are more serious; the fractured rib is coded and reported second.

16. A patient presents with leg pain and is referred for an x-ray to determine whether there is a fracture. During the performance of the diagnostic test, the interpreting physician noted arthritis in the ankle. The final diagnosis is sprained ankle. Which is the secondary condition?

    a. arthritis
    b. fracture
    c. leg pain
    d. sprained ankle

17. A patient had a colonoscopy performed, and the encounter was reported as a V code for screening. A code for benign polyp was also reported. Which statement best describes the situation?

    a. The diagnostic test (colonoscopy) was performed in the absence of signs or symptoms, and the polyp was discovered upon screening.
    b. The diagnostic test (colonoscopy) was performed in the absence of signs or symptoms.
    c. There was a qualified diagnosis of benign polyp, which was confirmed by the colonoscopy.
    d. There was a qualified diagnosis of benign polyp, which was not confirmed by the colonoscopy.

18. Which health care service includes both preventative and acute care, is often provided as outpatient care, and is referred to as the point of first contact?

    a. primary health care
    b. principal health care
    c. secondary health care
    d. tertiary health care

19. Ambulatory patients (or outpatients) are treated and released the same day and do not stay overnight in the hospital, which means that their maximum length of stay is:

    a. 23 hours.
    b. 23 hours, 59 minutes, and 59 seconds.
    c. 24 hours.
    d. 24 hours, 59 minutes, and 59 seconds.

20. Which are treated for urgent problems (e.g., trauma) and are either released the same day or admitted to the hospital as inpatients?

    a. ambulatory surgery patients
    b. clinic outpatients
    c. emergency patients
    d. referred outpatients

Chapter 7
HCPCS Level II National Coding System

1. The HCPCS level II national coding system:
   a. describes common medical services and supplies not classified in CPT.
   b. ensures the uniform reporting of diagnoses on submitted claims.
   c. has code descriptors that describe diagnoses, services, and procedures.
   d. is a reimbursement methodology for making coverage and payment determinations.

2. HCPCS level II national codes are:
   a. intended for use by all private and public health insurers.
   b. maintained by the AMA's Editorial Board, which makes decisions about additions, revisions, and deletions.
   c. sometimes replaced by HCPCS level II temporary codes.
   d. updated by CMS when necessary, without participation by the HCPCS National Panel.

3. HCPCS level II temporary codes are:
   a. deleted if not replaced by permanent codes by the HCPCS National Panel within five years.
   b. included as over 50 percent of the HCPCS level II codes.
   c. maintained by the CMS and other members of the HCPCS National Panel, independent of HCPCS level II permanent codes.
   d. updated once a year on January 1.

4. In which section of HCPCS level II would you locate codes for durable medical equipment (DME)-related supplies, accessories, maintenance, and repair?
   a. Administrative, Miscellaneous and Investigational (A9000–A9999)
   b. Durable Medical Equipment (E0100–E9999)
   c. Medical and Surgical Supplies (A4000–A8999)
   d. Outpatient PPS (C1000–C9999)

5. In which section of HCPCS level II would you locate a code for an office visit provided for the sole purpose of monitoring or changing drug prescriptions used in the treatment of mental psychoneurotic and personality disorders?
   a. Diagnostic Radiology Services (R0000–R5999)
   b. Medical Services (M0000–M0301)
   c. Pathology and Laboratory Services (P0000–P9999)
   d. Procedures/Professional Services (Temporary) (G0000–G9999)

6. In which section of HCPCS level II would you locate codes for chemistry, microbiology, and toxicology tests?
   a. Administrative, Miscellaneous and Investigational (A9000–A9999)
   b. Diagnostic Radiology Services (R0000–R5999)
   c. Pathology and Laboratory Services (P0000–P9999)
   d. Procedures/Professional Services (Temporary) (G0000–G9999)

7. In which section of HCPCS level II would you locate codes for exercise equipment, noncovered items and services, nonprescription drugs, and radiopharmaceutical diagnostic imaging agents?
   a. Administrative, Miscellaneous and Investigational (A9000–A9999)
   b. Diagnostic Radiology Services (R0000–R5999)
   c. Drugs Administered Other Than Oral Method (J0000–J9999)
   d. Durable Medical Equipment (E0100–E9999)

8. Which ensures that the provider will receive reimbursement from the patient in the event that medical necessity cannot be established for a procedure, service, or supply?
   a. advance beneficiary notice
   b. HCPCS level II modifiers
   c. *Medicare Carriers Manual* (MCM)
   d. *Medicare National Coverage Determinations Manual*

9. Where can you find clarification about local coverage determinations (LCDs)?
   a. DME MAC medical review policies
   b. *Medicare Benefit Policy Manual*
   c. *Medicare National Coverage Determinations Manual*
   d. *Medicare Program Integrity Manual*

10. Which procedures/services fall under the jurisdiction of the primary MAC only?
    a. dental procedures
    b. enteral and parenteral therapy
    c. hearing and vision services
    d. prosthetic and orthotic procedures

11. A diabetic patient received a J-cell alkaline replacement battery for her home blood glucose monitor.
    a. A4233   c. A4235
    b. A4234   d. A4236

12. A pediatric patient received 1 unit (100 calories) of enteral soy-based formula through a feeding tube, nutritionally complete with intact nutrients.
    a. B4102   c. B4159
    b. B4103   d. B4160

13. Heavy-duty wheelchair.
    a. K0001   c. K0006
    b. K0003   d. K0007

14. Non-removable longitudinal arch support (attached to shoe), left foot.
    a. L3070   c. L3090
    b. L3070-LT   d. L3090-LT

15. Halo procedure, cervical halo incorporated into Milwaukee-type orthosis.
    a. L0120   c. L0820
    b. L0810   d. L0830

16. Transportation of portable ECG to facility or location, per patient.
    a. R0080   c. R0075
    b. R0070   d. R0076

17. Home infusion therapy, peritoneal dialysis, administrative services.
    a. S9330   c. S9339
    b. S9338   d. S9353

18. Substance abuse services, skills development.
    a. H0047   c. T1010
    b. H2034   d. T1012

19. Assistive listening telecommunication device for the deaf (TDD).
    a. V5267   c. V5272
    b. V5269   d. V5273

20. Compression burn garment, chin strap, custom fabricated.
    a. A6501   c. A6504
    b. A6502   d. A6512

Chapter 8
Introduction to CPT Coding

1. The regulation that required new, revised, and deleted CPT codes to be implemented each January 1 was a result of the:
   a. American Medical Association CPT Editorial Board's publication of "early release" codes.
   b. Health Insurance, Portability, and Accountability Act (HIPAA).
   c. Medicare Prescription Drug, Improvement, and Modernization Act (MMA).
   d. Omnibus Budget Reconciliation Act (OBRA).

2. The draping and positioning of a patient is coded as:
   a. additions to the standard of practice.
   b. billable services.
   c. integral to the standard of practice.
   d. separately reportable services.

3. The code description for CPT code 70492:
   a. contains the entire description next to the code number.
   b. requires the coder to refer back to code 70490 for the common portion of the code description.
   c. requires the coder to report both codes 70492 and 70490.
   d. results in CPT code 70492 being considered a standalone code.

4. Using the CPT index, select the main term, subterm, and qualifier, respectively, that results in the assignment of a code for "transcatheter placement of an intracoronary stent(s), percutaneous, without therapeutic intervention; 2 vessels."
   a. insertion, stent, coronary
   b. percutaneous transluminal angioplasty, artery, coronary
   c. stent, placement, coronary
   d. transcatheter, stent, coronary

5. Using the CPT index, select the main term, subterm, and qualifier, respectively, that results in the assignment of a code for "liver imaging with vascular flow."
   a. hepatic duct, nuclear medicine, imaging
   b. imaging, liver
   c. liver, nuclear medicine, imaging
   d. vascular surgery, unlisted services and procedures

6. Code 45379 defines a colonoscopy with removal of foreign body. Using the CPT index, determine which main term would be used to locate that code.
   a. colon
   b. exploration
   c. foreign body removal
   d. removal

7. Appendix G contains a summary of CPT codes that include:
   a. add-on codes.
   b. conscious sedation.
   c. genetic testing modifiers.
   d. those exempt from modifier -51.

8. Which symbols identify CPT codes that are listed in its appendices?
   a. bullet, semicolon, bull's-eye
   b. plus, forbidden, bull's-eye
   c. plus, forbidden, bullet
   d. triangle, horizontal triangles, forbidden

165

9. A triangle symbol located to the left of a CPT code number signifies that the code is:
   a. new.
   b. reported with another code.
   c. revised.
   d. stand-alone.

10. Which symbol indicates that a change has been made to a CPT code, code description, guideline, and/or note when compared with the previous year's coding manual?
   a. bull's-eye
   b. forbidden
   c. semicolon
   d. triangle

11. Headings and subheadings are also called:
   a. categories and subcategories.
   b. main terms and subterms.
   c. sections and subsections.
   d. titles and subtitles.

12. Guidelines, notes, and descriptive qualifiers are found in CPT:
   a. headings only.
   b. sections and headings only.
   c. sections only.
   d. sections, subsections, headings, and subheadings.

13. "Radiology" and "Pathology and Laboratory" are CPT:
   a. descriptive qualifiers.
   b. headings.
   c. sections.
   d. subsections under the "laboratory" section of CPT.

14. If evaluation and management (E/M) services for a patient take longer than normal, which CPT modifier is added to the reported E/M code?
   a. -21
   b. -24
   c. -25
   d. -51

15. Terms found in provider documentation (e.g., difficult, extensive, or unusual) would support adding modifier _____ to a CPT code.
   a. -22
   b. -23
   c. -58
   d. -99

16. An intoxicated patient was brought to the emergency department with a skin laceration, for which he received stitches. The patient became combative and subsequently tore out the stitches, which were repaired by the same physician. Which CPT modifier would be reported for the second stitching procedure?
   a. -55
   b. -58
   c. -76
   d. -77

17. Which CPT modifier(s) are reported when surgery is performed by two surgeons?
   a. -58
   b. -62
   c. -76
   d. -77

18. Which CPT modifier is reported when a procedure is performed on an infant who weighs less than 4 kilograms (kg)?
   a. -54
   b. -59
   c. -63
   d. -66

19. NCCI edits are updated _____ and available to _____.
   a. annually; everyone
   b. annually; Medicare administrative contractors
   c. quarterly; everyone
   d. quarterly; physicians and other providers

20. The National Correct Coding Initiative (NCCI) edits are available as:
   a. paid subscriptions.
   b. paper-based document purchases.
   c. spreadsheets.
   d. telephone inquiry.

Chapter 9
CPT Evaluation and Management

1. Which code reflects a level 5 E/M service?
   a. 99211
   b. 99212
   c. 99214
   d. 99215

2. When an unlisted procedure or service code is reported, a special report must accompany the claim to describe _____ of the procedure or service.
   a. the nature, extent, and need
   b. the place of service and type of service
   c. the type of service and amount of time required
   d. whether the patient is new or established

3. Clinical examples of E/M codes are found in _____ of the CPT coding manual.
   a. Appendix A
   b. Appendix B
   c. Appendix C
   d. Appendix D

4. A patient returns to the physician's office today with neck and back pain. During a previous office visit last month, the patient was diagnosed as having multiple areas of bulging discs. The patient is not considered a surgical candidate at this time. Significant trauma in the past is noted, but C2-12 are intact. Deep tendon reflexes are within normal limits and symmetrical in the upper and lower extremities. Heart, lungs, and abdomen are without significant pathology. There are marked paravertebral spasms throughout the cervical, thoracic, and lumbar regions. HEENT: Patient has bilateral otitis externa noted. Which code is assigned for this level 4 E/M service?
   a. 99203
   b. 99204
   c. 99213
   d. 99214

5. Which terms describe the levels of work involved in medical decision-making?
   a. face-to-face, unit-floor, preencounter, postencounter
   b. minimal, self-limited, low severity, moderate severity, high severity
   c. problem focused, expanded problem focused, detailed, comprehensive
   d. straightforward, low complexity, moderate complexity, high complexity

6. A patient experiencing acute breathing trouble required one hour of direct face-to-face care from the physician. In addition to the appropriate level of E/M service code, which E/M subsection should be referenced to assign an additional code?
   a. Care Plan Oversight Services
   b. Case Management Services
   c. Preventive Medicine Services
   d. Prolonged Services

7. A physician spent approximately two hours on a conference call coordinating activities with members of a transplant team who were preparing to perform an organ transplant on his patient. From which E/M subsection would the code for this service be reported?
   a. Care Plan Oversight Services
   b. Case Management Services
   c. Critical Care Services
   d. Special Evaluation and Management Services

8. A patient was admitted to the hospital on November 4 for reconstructive surgery. After surgery, the physician reviewed the patient's record to determine how the patient was responding to the treatment. The patient was discharged November 6. Under which subsection of Hospital Inpatient Services would the code for the November 6 encounter be located?
   a. Hospital Discharge Services
   b. Initial Hospital Care
   c. Observation or Inpatient Care Services
   d. Subsequent Hospital Care

9. A patient presented with a bruised and swollen finger and was in extreme pain. The patient told the physician that she was loading groceries in her car when her son leaned on the door, causing it to slam shut on her finger. An x-ray was obtained, and the broken finger was put in a splint. After asking about any known allergies, the physician wrote a prescription for the pain and advised the patient to return if symptoms persisted beyond a week. Which type of history was performed?
   a. comprehensive
   b. detailed
   c. expanded problem focused
   d. problem focused

10. Which is considered a consultation and occurs when a surgeon requests that a specialist or another physician examine a patient and indicate whether the patient can withstand the expected risks of a specific surgery?
   a. confirmatory consultation
   b. physician standby services
   c. preoperative clearance
   d. special evaluation and management services

11. A woman is seen in the emergency department for a broken arm she sustained after slipping on ice. A problem focused history and physical were performed, and medical decision-making was straightforward.
   a. 99201
   b. 99221
   c. 99281
   d. 99282

12. A patient was seen in the office and underwent a baseline physical for the purpose of obtaining medical disability.
   a. 99201
   b. 99211
   c. 99381
   d. 99455

13. A patient is brought to the emergency department with a stab wound in the upper arm. An expanded problem focused history and examination are performed, and medical decision-making is of moderate complexity.
   a. 99202
   b. 99213
   c. 99232
   d. 99283

14. A patient with a heart condition is scheduled to undergo a cesarean section. Due to the high-risk nature of the delivery, the attending physician requests standby service from a cardiac surgeon; and 45 minutes later the patient delivers a healthy newborn with no complications.
   a. 99026
   b. 99027
   c. 99360
   d. 99360, 99360

15. An inpatient is seen for an initial consultation regarding a cardiac procedure. The consulting physician documented a comprehensive history and exam and spent 80 minutes with the patient. Medical decision-making was of moderate complexity.
   a. 99244
   b. 99254
   c. 99255
   d. 99274

16. An infant is admitted to the neonatal intensive care unit (NICU) shortly after birth on Tuesday morning. The infant remains on life support through Thursday.
   a. 99295, 99296, 99296
   b. 99468, 99469, 99469
   c. 99468
   d. 99468, 99469

17. A nursing facility resident began to experience periods of memory loss and disorientation. The physician performed a detailed interval history and exam. The physician spent 30 minutes talking with the patient and documenting in the medical record.
    a. 99307
    b. 99308
    c. 99309
    d. 99310

18. Dr. Killean called a patient to report the results of his blood test that was performed 10 days ago, and he instructed the patient to lower the dosage of his Coumadin and schedule an appointment to be seen in the office 30 days from now. Medical discussion during this telephone service was 10 minutes in duration.
    a. 99441
    b. 99442
    c. 99443
    d. 99444

19. Physician spent 40 minutes reviewing reports and modifying pain medication and oxygen orders for a 70-year-old hospice patient with terminal lung disease and a do-not-resuscitate order.
    a. 99374
    b. 99377
    c. 99378
    d. 99379

20. The physician documented the history and exam of a normal, healthy newborn admitted and discharged on the same day.
    a. 99461
    b. 99460
    c. 99463
    d. 99462

Chapter 10
CPT Anesthesia

1. Which is loss of pain sensation without loss of consciousness?
   - a. analgesia
   - b. analgesic
   - c. anesthesia
   - d. anesthetic

2. Which is the administration of varying amounts of local, regional, and certain mind-altering drugs during a procedure?
   - a. conscious sedation
   - b. general anesthesia
   - c. local anesthesia
   - d. monitored anesthesia care

3. The postanesthesia evaluation that is documented by the anesthesiologist or CRNA is _____.
   - a. also called postoperative pain management
   - b. done prior to the administration of anesthesia
   - c. included in the anesthesia services code
   - d. reported as a separate anesthesia service

4. When calculating anesthesia fees, which is the dollar amount assigned to a geographic location?
   - a. anesthesia conversion factor
   - b. anesthesia time unit(s)
   - c. base unit value
   - d. modifying unit

5. Which indicates the patient's condition at the time anesthesia was administered?
   - a. CPT alphabetic modifier
   - b. HCPCS level II modifier
   - c. physical status modifier
   - d. special report

6. Anesthesia services are reported based on time, which:
   - a. begins after the patient has received anesthesia and ends when the anesthesiologist or CRNA is no longer in personal attendance.
   - b. includes monitoring during administration of regional block anesthesia and during the procedure.
   - c. incorporates interval and recovery room times.
   - d. is reported in time units for which nonmonitored time is taken into consideration.

7. A diabetic patient who is otherwise healthy has a procedure performed under general anesthesia. The anesthesia services last 45 minutes, and the anesthesia code for this procedure has a base unit value of 5. The conversion factor for the geographic area is $19.20. Which is the correct formula for calculating the anesthesia fee?
   - a. $(5 + 3 + 1) \times \$19.20 = \$172.80$
   - b. $(5 + 45 + 1) \times \$19.20 = \$979.20$
   - c. $(\$19.20 + 3 + 1) \times 5 = \$116.00$
   - d. $(\$19.20 + 5 + 1) \times 3 = \$75.60$

8. Which anesthesia subsection contains the code(s) for surgery on the patella?
   - a. knee and popliteal area
   - b. pelvis (except hip)
   - c. perineum
   - d. shoulder and axilla

9. Which anesthesia subsection contains a code for lumbar hernia repair?
   - a. intrathoracic
   - b. lower abdomen
   - c. thorax
   - d. upper abdomen

10. Which anesthesia subsection contains the code(s) for myelography?
   - a. obstetric procedures
   - b. other procedures
   - c. radiological procedures
   - d. spine and spinal cord

11. An anesthesiologist provides anesthesia services for a right tympanotomy procedure performed on a healthy 6-month-old child.
   - a. 00126
   - b. 00126, 99100
   - c. 00126-P1-AA, 99100
   - d. 69420

12. A CRNA provides anesthesia services, with medical direction by a physician, for the reconstructive repair of pectus excavatum on a healthy patient.
   - a. 00474
   - b. 00474-P1-QX
   - c. 00474-P2
   - d. 21740

13. A CRNA provides monitored anesthesia care, without medical direction by a physician, during insertion of permanent transvenous pacemaker for a patient with pulmonary valve disorder.
   - a. 00530-P3
   - b. 00530-P3-QS-QZ
   - c. 00530-QS
   - d. 33206

14. An anesthesiologist provides anesthesia services for a lumbar sympathectomy on an otherwise healthy patient.
   - a. 00630-P1-AA
   - b. 00632-P1-AA
   - c. 00635-P1-AA
   - d. 32664

15. An anesthesiologist provides anesthesia services for a stomach restriction procedure on a patient with morbid obesity.
   - a. 00797
   - b. 00797-P1-AA
   - c. 00797-P2-AA
   - d. 00797-P3-AA

16. An anesthesiologist provides anesthesia services for a left femoral artery embolectomy procedure performed on a patient with an embolus in the left femoral artery (mild systemic disease).
   - a. 01270
   - b. 01272-P2-AA
   - c. 01274-P2-AA
   - d. 34201-P2-AA

17. A CRNA, with medical direction by a physician, provides anesthesia services to an otherwise healthy patient who undergoes an open elbow-to-shoulder tenotomy, left.
   - a. 01710
   - b. 01712-P1-QX
   - c. 01714
   - d. 23405-P1-QX

18. An anesthesiologist provides anesthesia services for a diagnostic arteriography of the left common carotid artery on a patient with possible carotid occlusion.
   - a. 01916-P2-AA
   - b. 01924-P2-AA
   - c. 01926-P2-AA
   - d. 01930-P2-AA

19. An anesthesiologist provides anesthesia services to a healthy patient who undergoes neuraxial labor anesthesia for planned vaginal delivery.
   - a. 01967
   - b. 01967-23
   - c. 01967-P1-AA
   - d. 01967-P1-23-AA

20. An anesthesiologist provides anesthesia services to a patient with type 1 diabetes mellitus who undergoes transurethral resection of a bladder tumor.
   - a. 00910-P2-AA
   - b. 00912-P2-AA
   - c. 00912-P3-AA
   - d. 52500-P3-AA

Chapter 11
CPT Surgery I

1. Which is true about the CPT code descriptions?
   a. CPT code descriptions do not include the numerous activities integral to the procedure, such as the administration of local anesthesia and the initial incision.
   b. CPT code descriptions include all activities integral to the procedure.
   c. If an activity is not listed in the code description, it should be coded separately.
   d. The information in each code description contains all of the information necessary to select the proper code.

2. Which term describes the ablation of benign, premalignant, or malignant tissues by any method?
   a. destruction
   b. excision
   c. removal
   d. repair

3. The CMS national definition for a global surgical package:
   a. categorizes surgeries as major or minor and establishes a postoperative global period for each surgical procedure.
   b. ensures Medicare payments for services that are less comprehensive than intended.
   c. ensures Medicare payments for services that are more comprehensive than intended.
   d. ensures that payments are made consistently for the same services by all third-party payers across the nation.

4. Add-on codes:
   a. allow physicians to bundle procedures and services performed at the same time as the primary procedure.
   b. are usually reported as stand-alone codes because they are performed in addition to another procedure.
   c. can be identified by specific language in the code descriptor, such as "each additional" or "list separately in addition to primary procedure."
   d. sometimes qualify for the multiple procedure concept, which means that modifier -51 must be added to the CPT code.

5. CPT code descriptions that contain the phrase "separate procedure" in parentheses:
   a. are always performed as a separate procedure or service.
   b. are always performed as an integral component of a total service or procedure.
   c. are commonly performed as an integral component of a total service or procedure.
   d. are reported as an additional procedure when performed during the same operative episode as a more comprehensive procedure.

6. During the global period:
   a. complications subsequent to surgery are not reimbursed by the payer.
   b. distinct surgical procedures performed to treat complications during the postoperative period are not reported.
   c. normal, uncomplicated care provided by the surgeon who performed the original procedure is not coded or reported separately.
   d. the surgeon who performed the original procedure reports evaluation and management codes for normal, uncomplicated care.

7. During fine-needle aspiration, imaging guidance is typically used when the cyst or mass is not _____.
   a. malignant
   b. palpable
   c. small
   d. visible

8. Wound repair is coded with the appropriate evaluation and management code when the sole repair material used includes _____.
   a. adhesive strips
   b. staples
   c. sutures
   d. tissue adhesives

9. A biopsy was performed on a woman who did not have an established diagnosis. The results of the biopsy would determine whether to perform a mastectomy. Which is the correct way to report the biopsy?
   a. The biopsy code is not reported.
   b. The biopsy code is separately reported, and modifier -58 may be added to indicate that the biopsy and mastectomy are staged or planned procedures.
   c. The biopsy is coded and separately reported. Modifier -59 may be used appropriately to indicate that the biopsy and the mastectomy are distinct procedural services.
   d. The biopsy is separately reported. Modifier -78 may be used appropriately to indicate a return to the operating room for a related procedure during the postoperative period.

10. Complex repair of 8.5 cm wound, scalp, with extensive debridement of contaminated skin and subcutaneous tissue.
    a. 13121
    b. 13122
    c. 13121, 13122
    d. 13121, 13122, 11042

11. Excision of 1.5 cm malignant lesion, left ear. Incision and drainage performed to access lesion. Intermediate repair of excision site performed.
    a. 10060-LT, 11642-LT
    b. 11642-LT
    c. 11642-LT, 12031-LT
    d. 11642-LT, 12051-LT

12. Removal of four benign lesions from trunk, each 1.0 cm in size including margins. Simple repair performed.
    a. 11406
    b. 11400, 12002-51
    c. 11401, 11401-59, 11401-59, 11401-59
    d. 11406, 12002-51

13. Adjacent tissue transfer of 3.2 sq cm defect, scalp, after removal of 3.2 cm lesion performed during the same operative session.
    a. 11404, 14000
    b. 14000
    c. 14020
    d. 14020, 11404

14. Bilateral blepharoplasty of upper eyelids.
    a. 15820-50
    b. 15822-50
    c. 15821
    d. 15822

15. Patient presents to the emergency department with multiple lacerations. Simple repair was performed on 7.9 cm laceration of right leg, 6 cm laceration of right arm, 4 cm laceration of right cheek, and 2.5 cm laceration of right ear.
    a. 12002, 12004-51, 12014-51
    b. 12002, 12004, 12013, 12013
    c. 12005, 12013-51
    d. 12005, 12014-51

16. Incision and drainage of three cysts, right buttock.
    a. 10040
    b. 10060
    c. 10061
    d. 10080

17. Escharotomy of chest, three incisions.
    a. 16035
    b. 16036
    c. 16035, 16036
    d. 16035, 16036, 16036

18. Patient underwent 30 minutes of electrolysis.
    a. 17340
    b. 17360
    c. 17380
    d. 17999

19. Bilateral removal of intact mammary implants.
    a. 19316
    b. 19318-50
    c. 19324-50
    d. 19328-50

20. Patient underwent simple repair of the scalp (1.5 centimeters) and face (1.0 centimeter).
    a. 12001, 12011
    b. 12002
    c. 12013
    d. 12032

Chapter 12
CPT Surgery II

1. Codes 20900–20938 are reported when _____ tissue (originating in the patient's body) is obtained through separate skin or fascial incisions.
   a. allogenous
   b. autogenous
   c. osteogenesis
   d. rhytides

2. A patient suffered a traumatic amputation in an accident and underwent replantation surgery. A code from the range 20802–20838 was reported. Which procedures are reported with codes in this range?
   a. arthrodesis, cleansing, and debridement
   b. arthrodesis, cleansing, and internal fixation
   c. arthrodesis, cleansing, debridement, internal fixation, and repair of tendons
   d. internal fixation and repair of tendons

3. A surgeon performed an osteotomy and bone graft during the same operative session. Which CPT coding rule applies?
   a. Do not report a separate code for the osteotomy.
   b. Do not report a separate code for the bone graft.
   c. Add modifier -51 (Multiple Procedure) to the bone graft code.
   d. Do not add modifier -51 (Multiple Procedure) to the bone graft code.

4. Which are bundled in the tendon repair codes?
   a. application of immobilization, extension of the excision, and repair and closure of tendon sheath
   b. application of immobilization, repair of nerves or arteries, and repair and closure of tendon sheath
   c. extension of the excision, harvesting and inserting tendon grafts from another site, and repairing nerves or arteries
   d. harvesting and inserting tendon grafts from another site, repairing nerves or arteries, and treating fractures

5. The Pelvis and Hip Joint heading in the Musculoskeletal System subsection includes codes for procedures performed on the:
   a. femur and its tibial plateau.
   b. femur and popliteal bone.
   c. head and neck of the femur.
   d. head, neck, and tibial plateau of the femur.

6. Conversion of previous hip surgery to total hip arthroplasty, left side.
   a. 27130-LT
   b. 27132-LT
   c. 27134-LT
   d. 27137-LT

7. Arthrocentesis was performed for injection of medication, left acromioclavicular joint, for pain relief.
   a. 20600-LT
   b. 20605-LT
   c. 23044-LT
   d. 23130-LT

8. Arthroscopy of the right ankle with fusion of the tibiotalar and fibulotalar joints.
   a. 29894-RT
   b. 29894-RT, 29899-51-RT
   c. 29894-RT, 29899-RT
   d. 29899-RT

9. A 21-year-old male presented to the emergency department with pain in the right hand that began when he pounded his desk this morning after an argument with his boss. He was diagnosed with nondisplaced

fractures of the 3rd and 4th right metacarpals. A cast was applied, and the patient was instructed to take Tylenol for pain.

a. 26600-F7

b. 26600-F7, 26600-F8

c. 26600-F7, 26600-51-F8, 29085

d. 26600-F8, 29085

10. Bilateral reconstruction of medial collateral ligament, elbow, with tendon graft.

a. 24344-50

b. 24345-50

c. 24346-50

d. 24360-50

11. Three bony plates are located on each side of the entrance to the nasal cavity. These bony plates and the entrance to the nasal cavity are called, respectively, the:

a. nasal vestibules and septum.

b. nasal vestibules and turbinates.

c. septum and nasal vestibule.

d. turbinates and nasal vestibule.

12. When diagnostic endoscopy is performed, administration of local anesthesia and electrocautery are bundled in the reported code, in addition to access to:

a. different cavities and extensive shaving/debridement.

b. different cavities and some shaving/debridement.

c. one cavity and extensive shaving/debridement.

d. one cavity and some shaving/debridement.

13. In which situation is a laryngoscopy procedure code separately reported?

a. diagnostic laryngoscopy only

b. endotracheal tube for nonemergent reasons

c. endotracheal tube to provide air passage in an emergency situation

d. tracheostomy

14. Endoscopy codes 31622–31629 are reported to:

a. describe multiple procedures performed and reported with codes 31622–31629. (Each code is reported separately, and modifier -51 is added to the subsequent codes.)

b. describe procedures in codes 31622–31629 that are not distinct surgical procedures and that are considered integral components of one another.

c. describe procedures that involve use of a bronchoscope, with or without fluoroscopic guidance, to visualize all major lobar and segmental bronchi.

d. indicate that these procedures do not include obtaining diagnostic specimens as part of the examination.

15. Which is the removal of a portion of lung that is less than a segment?

a. lobectomy

b. pneumocentesis

c. segmentectomy

d. wedge resection

16. A patient underwent surgical sinus endoscopy on the left frontal sinus. Sinusotomy and diagnostic endoscopy of the left frontal sinus were also performed.

a. 31070-LT, 31231-LT

b. 31276-LT

c. 31276-LT, 31070-LT, 31231-LT

d. 31276-LT, 31231-LT

17. Bilateral sinusotomy of the frontal, maxillary, and sphenoid sinuses.

a. 31070, 31020-51, 31050-51

b. 31070-50, 31020-50, 31050-50

c. 31090-50

d. 31090-50-51

18. Partial anterovertical laryngectomy.

a. 31370

b. 31375

c. 31380

d. 31382

19. Excision of tracheal tumor using cervical approach.

a. 31750

b. 31781

c. 31785

d. 31786

20. Surgical thoracoscopy with excision of pericardial mass.

a. 32650

b. 32658

c. 32661

d. 32662

Chapter 13
CPT Surgery III

1. Selective vascular catheterization procedures require separate coding of the:
   a. administration of local anesthesia.
   b. diagnostic procedure and/or therapeutic procedure as well as vascular access.
   c. introduction of the needle or catheter as well as vascular access.
   d. introduction of the needle or catheter or injection of contrast material.

2. Which procedure describes the insertion of a needle to withdraw fluid from the pericardial sac?
   a. pericardiectomy
   b. pericardiocentesis
   c. pericardiotomy
   d. tube pericardiostomy

3. Which is the medical term for the resultant backflow of blood when two valvular flaps do not close properly?
   a. achalasia
   b. atresia
   c. prolapse
   d. stenosis

4. Which is coded as congenital heart defect?
   a. aneurysm
   b. cardiac tumor
   c. coronary arteriovenous fistula
   d. truncus arteriosus

5. When a patient's coronary arteries contain extensive cholesterol plaque, a coronary artery bypass graft (CABG) procedure cannot be performed until the plaque is removed via:
   a. cardiac ablation.
   b. commissurotomy.
   c. coronary endarterectomy.
   d. transmyocardial revascularization.

6. Which is the excision of plaque from inside a blood vessel that involves puncturing the artery with a large needle and inserting a guidewire into the artery?
   a. open transluminal angioplasty
   b. open transluminal atherectomy
   c. percutaneous transluminal angioplasty
   d. percutaneous transluminal atherectomy

7. Bone marrow needle biopsy, right femur.
   a. 38220
   b. 38221
   c. 38230
   d. 38240

8. Transcatheter procedure code 37204 was performed on two vessels from one anatomic structure and another vessel in a different anatomic structure. Which is the correct way to report code 37204 for this procedure?
   a. 37204, 37204
   b. 37204, 37204, 37204
   c. 37204, 37204-59
   d. 37204-51

9. Add-on codes 35685–35686 describe additional procedures or techniques that may be required during a lower extremity bypass graft procedure. They are performed to improve the open and unblocked status of a blood vessel of lower extremity synthetic or autogenous arterial bypass grafts. The terms for the additional procedures and the open and unblocked status are, respectively:
   a. adjacent techniques and patency
   b. adjacent techniques and tunneled
   c. adjuvant techniques and patency
   d. adjuvant techniques and tunneled

10. Which two types of stem cells are located in bone marrow?
    a. hemopoietic and stromal
    b. implanted and tunneled
    c. red and white
    d. red and yellow

11. Transmyocardial laser revascularization, by thoracotomy, performed during pulmonary valve replacement.
    a. 33140, 33475
    b. 33475
    c. 33475, 33140, 33141
    d. 33475, 33141

12. Patient underwent insertion of dual-chamber pacing cardioverter-defibrillator. A left ventricle lead was placed for biventricular pacing.
    a. 33216, 33225-51
    b. 33217
    c. 33217, 33225
    d. 33217, 33225-51

13. Operative incision and reconstruction of atria for treatment of atrial flutter (Maze procedure).
    a. 33250
    b. 33251
    c. 33255
    d. 33261

14. Repair of anomalous coronary artery by graft, with endarterectomy, without cardiopulmonary bypass.
    a. 33503
    b. 33503, 33572
    c. 33504
    d. 33504, 33572

15. Shunt procedure performed from the superior vena cava to the pulmonary artery, with flow to both lungs.
    a. 33750
    b. 33755
    c. 33766
    d. 33767

16. One segment of artery harvested from left arm (for coronary artery bypass graft surgery).
    a. 33508-LT
    b. 35500-LT
    c. 35572-LT
    d. 35600-LT

17. Patient returned to surgery for exploration of postoperative hemorrhage in abdomen.
    a. 35800
    b. 35840
    c. 35840-76
    d. 35840-78

18. Percutaneous carotid catheterization and arteriogram were performed on right side to confirm the need for carotid stenting. The patient then underwent transcatheter placement of an intravascular stent in the right cervical carotid artery, percutaneous, with distal embolic protection.
    a. 36620-RT, 37216-RT
    b. 37215-RT
    c. 37215-RT, 36620-RT
    d. 37216-RT

19. Direct open arteriovenous anastomosis.
    a. 36810
    b. 36821
    c. 36825
    d. 36830

20. A 30-year-old patient underwent repair of acute traumatic diaphragmatic hernia.
    a. 39503
    b. 39520
    c. 39540
    d. 39541

Chapter 14
CPT Surgery IV

1. Which level of lip repair is assigned a code from the Digestive System subsection rather than the Integumentary System subsection?
   - a. complex
   - b. full-thickness
   - c. intermediate
   - d. layered

2. Codes for glossectomy procedures are assigned from the _____ heading of the Digestive System subsection.
   - a. Dentoalveolar Structures
   - b. Palate and Uvula
   - c. Tongue and Floor of Mouth
   - d. Vestibule of Mouth

3. How is hemorrhage control following a tonsillectomy and adenoidectomy procedure reported?
   - a. Do not report a separate code because hemorrhage control is included in the tonsillectomy and adenoidectomy procedure codes.
   - b. Report a code for hemorrhage control following tonsillectomy and adenoidectomy procedures and add modifier -59 to that code.
   - c. Report a code for the tonsillectomy or adenoidectomy procedure and add modifier -78.
   - d. Report a separate code for hemorrhage control following tonsillectomy and adenoidectomy procedures and add modifier -78 to the code.

4. When documentation indicates that enterolysis was extensive and added significantly to the other major procedure performed, report enterolysis code 44005 (freeing of intestinal adhesions) followed by modifier:
   - a. -22
   - b. -51
   - c. -59
   - d. -76

5. Bladder irrigation code 51700 is reported:
   - a. for irrigation as an independent therapeutic service.
   - b. for irrigation with therapeutic agents or for irrigation as an independent therapeutic service.
   - c. when performed during a more comprehensive procedure.
   - d. when performed to access or visualize the urinary system.

6. Code 44955 is reported for an appendectomy when it is performed _____.
   - a. as the primary procedure
   - b. during intra-abdominal surgery
   - c. for a ruptured appendix with abscess or generalized peritonitis
   - d. for an indicated purpose during the same operative session as another major procedure

7. The percutaneous drainage of a liver abscess (47011) includes _____.
   - a. final removal of the catheter
   - b. initial insertion of the catheter
   - c. radiologic guidance
   - d. final removal of the catheter, initial insertion of the catheter, and radiologic guidance

8. A patient underwent the surgical treatment of an anal fistula, which required a submuscular fistulectomy. Which description would be documented in the operative report?
   - a. excision of multiple fistulas
   - b. removal of an anal fistula, including division of the sphincter muscle
   - c. removal of an anal fistula, without division of the sphincter muscle
   - d. use of a seton to cut through the fistula

181

9. When multiple endoscopic approaches are performed to accomplish the same procedure, report a code for:

    a. each endoscopic approach performed, adding modifier -51 to each less extensive code.

    b. each endoscopic approach performed.

    c. the least extensive code only.

    d. the successful endoscopic approach only.

10. Urethral catheterization codes (51701–51702) are reported when urethral catheterization is:

    a. necessary for urethral dilation and for accomplishment of a more extensive procedure.

    b. necessary to accomplish a more extensive procedure.

    c. performed independently of another procedure.

    d. performed preceding the scheduled surgery.

11. Diaphragmatic hernia repair performed on neonate.

    a. 39502   c. 39540-63

    b. 39503   d. 39541-63

12. Laser-assisted uvulopalatoplasty, second treatment session.

    a. 42145   c. 42299

    b. 42145-51   d. 42299, 42299

13. Diagnostic endoscopic retrograde cholangiopancreatography (ERCP) with washing and collection of specimens.

    a. 43260   c. 43264

    b. 43261   d. 43269

14. Bilateral posterior vestibuloplasty.

    a. 40840   c. 40843

    b. 40842-50   d. 40845

15. Suture of small intestine for perforated ulcer.

    a. 44602   c. 44604

    b. 44603   d. 44605

16. Partial proctectomy with anastomosis using transsacral approach.

    a. 45110   c. 45113

    b. 45111   d. 45116

17. Donor hepatectomy from cadaver.

    a. 47133   c. 47141

    b. 47140   d. 47142

18. Repair of strangulated initial inguinal hernia, 1-year-old child.

    a. 49501   c. 49521

    b. 49507   d. 49520

19. Laparoscopic partial nephrectomy.

    a. 50240   c. 50545

    b. 50543   d. 50548

20. Aspiration of bladder with insertion of suprapubic catheter with ultrasonic guidance.

    a. 51100, 76942   c. 51102, 77012

    b. 51101, 77012   d. 51102, 76942

Chapter 15
CPT Surgery V

1. Which is the abnormal dilation of the spermatic cord veins in the scrotum?
   - a. BPH
   - b. orchiopexy
   - c. TULIP
   - d. varicocele

2. Which is included in the delivery service and is therefore not coded and reported separately?
   - a. admission to the hospital for observation prior to delivery
   - b. delivery of the placenta
   - c. treatment of postpartum medical complications
   - d. tubal ligation performed after delivery

3. The Endocrine System subsection includes procedures performed on the endocrine glands and the:
   - a. carotid body.
   - b. pineal glands.
   - c. pituitary gland.
   - d. carotid body and pineal and pituitary glands.

4. Which causes carpal tunnel syndrome?
   - a. compression of the median nerve at the wrist
   - b. numbness, pain, and weakness in the hand and wrist
   - c. repetitive flexing and extension of the wrist
   - d. thickening of the protective sheaths that surround each of the tendons

5. Which is the removal of a portion of the vertebra and adjacent intervertebral disks?
   - a. corpectomy
   - b. diskectomy
   - c. laminectomy
   - d. osteophytectomy

6. During a spinal procedure, an incision is made into the area of the affected vertebral segment and the incision is inferiorly curved out to the lateral plane. Paraspinous muscles are mobilized medially (denervating and devascularizing these structures). The muscles are lifted from the spinous process; and they are divided and lifted from the ribs, exposing the vertebral segment. Which surgical approach has been performed?
   - a. anterolateral approach
   - b. costovertebral approach
   - c. lateral extracavitary approach
   - d. transpedicular approach

7. Which procedure, classified in the Eye and Ocular Adnexa subsection, includes severing and removing the eyeball from extraorbital muscles and the optic nerve?
   - a. enucleation of the eye
   - b. evisceration of ocular contents
   - c. exenteration of the orbit
   - d. extracapsular cataract extraction

8. A common procedure performed to repair facial nerve damage is total nerve decompression, which is used to treat symptoms of:
   - a. Bell's palsy.
   - b. carpal tunnel syndrome.
   - c. orbital implants.
   - d. strabismus.

9. An operating microscope is reported in addition to the primary surgical procedure for:
   - a. all encounters during which an operating microscope is used.
   - b. performance of microsurgery techniques.
   - c. procedures where use of an operating microscope is an inclusive component.
   - d. visualization with a magnifying loupe or corrected vision.

10. Which involves the removal of skin and deep subcutaneous tissue?
    a. laser ablation of the vulva   c. simple vulvectomy
    b. radical vulvectomy   d. volvulus

11. Bilateral epididymovasostomy requiring use of operating microscope.
    a. 54900, 69990   c. 54901
    b. 54900-50   d. 54901, 69990

12. Vaginal closure of vesicovaginal fistula; concomitant cystotomy with drainage.
    a. 57310   c. 57320, 51040
    b. 57320   d. 57330

13. Patient returns to physician for normal postpartum care after uncomplicated pregnancy, obstetric care, and vaginal delivery using forceps.
    a. 59400   c. 59410
    b. 59409   d. 59430

14. Complete thyroidectomy.
    a. 60220   c. 60252
    b. 60240   d. 60260

15. Patient with craniosynostosis underwent craniectomy that required a single cranial suture.
    a. 61550   c. 61556
    b. 61552   d. 61558

16. Extradural excision of vascular lesion of infratemporal fossa with repair by anastomosis.
    a. 61605   c. 61606
    b. 61605, 61610   d. 61607

17. Patient with intracranial lesion underwent creation of burr hole and stereotactic biopsy.
    a. 61140   c. 61750
    b. 61140, 61750   d. 61750, 61140

18. Patient with glaucoma underwent sector iridectomy with corneoscleral section.
    a. 66625   c. 66635
    b. 66630   d. 66680

19. Removal of superficial foreign body from the conjunctiva of the external eye.
    a. 65205   c. 65220
    b. 65210   d. 65222

20. Patient underwent tympanoplasty with mastoidectomy and tympanic membrane repair.
    a. 69641   c. 69642
    b. 69641, 69610   d. 69643

Chapter 16
CPT Radiology

1. *Coronal, midsagittal, sagittal,* and *transverse* are terms that describe:
   a. components of radiology procedures.
   b. contrast agents.
   c. planes of view.
   d. radiographic projections.

2. Which modifiers are commonly added to radiology codes to indicate the component provided?
   a. -26 and -TC
   b. -50 and -51
   c. -52 and -76
   d. -LT and -RT

3. Component coding:
   a. allows for the reporting of a radiology procedure code and a surgical procedure code to completely describe the service provided.
   b. combines the technical and professional components into a single code.
   c. indicates that a provider owns the equipment and performs both the technical and professional components.
   d. requires that modifier -52 be added to the radiology code reported.

4. Which includes standard radiographs, contrast studies, computed tomography (CT), and magnetic resonance imaging (MRI)?
   a. interventional diagnostic imaging
   b. invasive diagnostic imaging
   c. noninvasive diagnostic imaging
   d. nuclear imaging

5. Which identifies nerve construction or inflammation and the degree of fluid flow in the epidural space?
   a. computed tomography
   b. epidurography
   c. magnetic resonance angiography
   d. mammography

6. A separate code is reported for:
   a. an intrathecal injection.
   b. diagnostic angiography or venography (radiologic supervision and interpretation).
   c. therapeutic nuclear medicine procedures.
   d. therapeutic transcatheter radiologic supervision and interpretation.

7. Which radiologic procedure involves x-rays of different angles to create cross-sectional images of organs, bones, and tissues to visualize blood flow in arterial and venous vessels throughout the body?
   a. computed axial tomography
   b. computed tomography angiography
   c. magnetic resonance angiography
   d. magnetic resonance imaging

8. Amplitude modulation, gray-scale ultrasound, motion mode, and real-time scan are:
   a. planes of view for radiology procedures.
   b. radiographic projections.
   c. types of ophthalmic ultrasound.
   d. ultrasound display modes.

9. Types of radiation oncology treatment devices include:
   a. blocks, breast boards, wedges, and eye shields.
   b. neutron beam and proton beam.

c. therapeutic port film and megaelectron volts.

d. treatment volume determination, treatment time/dosage determination, and choice of treatment modality.

10. A patient underwent a procedure that measures thyroid function to determine how much iodine the thyroid absorbs. The type of procedure that the patient had is a(n):

a. photon absorptiometry.

b. tomographic single photon emission computed tomography.

c. uptake test.

d. vascular flow exam.

11. After being tackled in a football game, a patient with complaints of pain and trouble breathing underwent rib x-rays on both sides. Three views were obtained.

a. 71100   c. 71110

b. 71100-51   d. 71110-50

12. Myelography of the cervical and thoracic spine, radiological supervision and interpretation.

a. 72240, 72255   c. 72270-51

b. 72270   d. 72270-52

13. Magnetic resonance imaging of thigh with contrast.

a. 73718   c. 73722

b. 73719   d. 73725

14. Intravenous (IV) urography with tomography, professional component.

a. 74400   c. 74400-26, 74150

b. 74400-26   d. 74410-26

15. Angiography of right cervical carotid artery.

a. 75671-RT   c. 75680-RT

b. 75676-RT   d. 75685-RT

16. A patient in the twentieth week of her pregnancy underwent transabdominal uterine ultrasound, real time with image documentation, for fetal and maternal evaluation, single gestation.

a. 76801   c. 76805

b. 76802   d. 76810

17. Therapeutic radiology treatment planning with simulation of a single treatment area and no blocking.

a. 77261   c. 77263

b. 77262   d. 77299

18. Pulmonary perfusion imaging, particulate, with ventilation imaging, aerosol, one or multiple projections.

a. 78580   c. 78585

b. 78584   d. 78588

19. Radiopharmaceutical therapy, intravenous administration.

a. 79005   c. 79440

b. 79101   d. 79445

20. Patient underwent magnetic resonance imaging (MRI) of neck without contrast, followed by imaging with contrast.

a. 70542, 70540   c. 70547, 70548

b. 70543   d. 70549

Chapter 17
CPT Pathology and Laboratory

1. A patient presents with a variety of symptoms for which blood tests are ordered. In the lab, venipuncture is performed. Because the vein collapses prior to completion, a second needle is placed in a different vein. A total of three separate color-coded vials of blood are drawn and labeled for testing. How many codes are reported for specimen collection?
   a. none
   b. one
   c. two
   d. three

2. Which are proteins in the body that are made by the immune system and that fight infection and disease?
   a. adjuvants
   b. analytes
   c. antibodies
   d. antigens

3. A Medicare patient has tests performed at a lab that has a CLIA waiver. Which HCPCS level II modifier is added to pathology and laboratory service codes?
   a. -59
   b. -P1
   c. -QW
   d. -TC

4. The unit of pathology service is a(n):
   a. assay.
   b. block.
   c. section.
   d. specimen.

5. A patient is seen for blood work; and a panel that is performed includes CBC, automated Hgb, Hct, RBC, WBC, and platelet count (85027). Later that day a separate hemoglobin test is run (85018). The coder reports 85027 and 85018-91. Under which condition is it appropriate to report both codes?
   a. Multiple tests are performed as part of a series.
   b. The original panel produces an abnormal hemoglobin result.
   c. The test is repeated due to technician error.
   d. An equipment malfunction occurred during the performance of the test.

6. Organ or disease-oriented panels:
   a. may be reported in addition to individual codes for each lab test performed.
   b. may be reported when most of the component tests have been performed.
   c. were developed for coding purposes only.
   d. were developed for use as clinical parameters.

7. In addition to the Drug Testing and the Therapeutic Drug Assays subsections of pathology and laboratory, CPT codes reported for drug testing are also located in the _____ subsection.
   a. Chemistry
   b. Hematology and Coagulation
   c. Immunology
   d. Urinalysis

8. Test panels from the _____ subsection include the administration of agents that cause production of hormones or other secretions.
   a. Anatomic Pathology
   b. Evocative/Suppression
   c. Immunology
   d. Microbiology

9. Which is the study of microbes?
   a. cytopathology
   b. hematology
   c. immunology
   d. microbiology

187

10. Which CPT Pathology and Laboratory subsection codes are reported for physician services only?
    a. Anatomic Pathology
    b. Cytogenetic Studies
    c. Organ or Disease-Oriented Panels
    d. Surgical Pathology

11. Glucose tolerance test, six specimens.
    a. 82951
    b. 82951, 82952
    c. 82951, 82951-91
    d. 82951, 82952, 82952, 82952

12. Bilirubin test from feces specimen.
    a. 82247
    b. 82248
    c. 82252
    d. 82270

13. Breath specimen analyzed for urease activity in Helicobacter pylori, nonradioactive isotope.
    a. 83009
    b. 83013
    c. 83014
    d. 87338

14. Mutation identification by sequencing, one segment, via molecular diagnostics.
    a. 83903
    b. 83904
    c. 83905
    d. 83906

15. Qualitative analysis of porphyrins in urine.
    a. 84119
    b. 84120
    c. 84126
    d. 84127

16. Manual leukocyte cell count, repeated later in the same day for comparison.
    a. 85032
    b. 85032, 85032-51
    c. 85032, 85032-91
    d. 85048, 85048-91

17. Complete semen analysis, including volume, count, motility, and differential.
    a. 89300
    b. 89310
    c. 89320
    d. 89321

18. Blood culture for bacteria, with isolation and presumptive identification of isolates.
    a. 87040
    b. 87045
    c. 87046
    d. 87075

19. Surgical pathology, gross examination only.
    a. 88300
    b. 88302
    c. 88304
    d. 88305

20. Patient with adrenal insufficiency underwent ACTH stimulation panel including cortisol × 2.
    a. 80400
    b. 80402
    c. 80412
    d. 82024

Chapter 18
CPT Medicine

1. Upon review of ventilator management codes 94002–94005, the note states that these codes are not reported with codes:
   a. 00100–01999
   b. 10021–69990
   c. 99201–99499
   d. 90281–99607

2. Acupuncture is classified in _____-minute increments of face-to-face patient contact.
   a. 10
   b. 15
   c. 20
   d. 30

3. An immune globulin:
   a. contains antigens.
   b. is administered as immunization against infectious agents.
   c. provides long-term protection against infectious agents.
   d. provides temporary protection against infectious agents.

4. Under which heading is the flash symbol found?
   a. Evaluation and Management
   b. Immune Globulins
   c. Immunization Administration for Vaccines/Toxoids
   d. Vaccines/Toxoids

5. Which typically includes a system of desensitization?
   a. behavior-modifying psychotherapy
   b. interactive psychotherapy
   c. psychodynamic psychotherapy
   d. supportive psychotherapy

6. A patient receives ongoing psychotherapy services from a psychologist at a facility and occasionally has an evaluation and management encounter with the resident psychiatrist to evaluate her prescribed medications. When reporting services for this patient, the pharmacologic management service is:
   a. coded and reported separately by the psychiatrist.
   b. coded and reported separately by the psychologist.
   c. included in psychotherapy services reported by the psychologist.
   d. included in the evaluation and management service reported by the psychiatrist.

7. Which service performed during cardiac catheterization is reported separately?
   a. cardiac output measurement
   b. fluoroscopic guidance procedure codes classified by CPT as supervision and interpretation
   c. imaging supervision, interpretation, and documented report for injection procedures
   d. injection procedures during cardiac catheterization

8. Codes for cerebrovascular arterial studies are found in which Medicine subsection?
   a. Cardiovascular
   b. Neurology and Neuromuscular Procedures
   c. Noninvasive Vascular Diagnostic Studies
   d. Pulmonary

9. Which type(s) of allergy sensitivity test(s) identify allergies to insect venom and penicillin?
   a. epicutaneous
   b. intracutaneous
   c. percutaneous and epicutaneous
   d. percutaneous and intracutaneous

189

10. Which Medicine subsection contains codes for sleep testing?
   a. Biofeedback
   b. Neurology and Neuromuscular Procedures
   c. Other Services and Procedures
   d. Psychiatry

11. End-stage renal disease (ESRD) services for 17-year-old patient with one face-to-face physician visit per month.
   a. 90953   c. 90958
   b. 90957   d. 90959

12. Manometric study for gastric motility.
   a. 91010   c. 91020
   b. 91012   d. 91022

13. Percutaneous transluminal coronary balloon angioplasty of one vessel.
   a. 92982   c. 92986
   b. 92984   d. 92987

14. Under moderate sedation, a patient underwent transesophageal echocardiography in real time with 2D image documentation, including probe placement, image acquisition, interpretation, and report.
   a. 93312   c. 93313
   b. 93312, 99143   d. 93318, 99143

15. Patient with acute airway obstruction received two pressurized inhalation treatments.
   a. 94640   c. 94640, 94640-51
   b. 94640, 94640-76   d. 94640-76

16. Needle electromyography of both arms and both legs.
   a. 95860   c. 95863
   b. 95861   d. 95864

17. Intra-arterial chemotherapy administration, infusion technique, one hour.
   a. 96409   c. 96420
   b. 96413   d. 96422

18. Five hours of work hardening/conditioning.
   a. 97545, 97546   c. 97545, 97546, 97546, 97546
   b. 97546, 97546-51   d. 97545, 97546, 97546-51

19. A patient received extraspinal manipulation on four regions from a chiropractor.
   a. 98926   c. 98943
   b. 98941   d. 98943, 98943, 98943, 98943

20. A therapist administered oxygen therapy to a patient in the patient's home.
   a. 99183   c. 99504
   b. 99503   d. 99509

Chapter 19
Insurance and Reimbursement

1. Which of the following eliminated carriers, fiscal intermediaries (FIs), and durable medical equipment regional carriers (DMERCs) and created MACs?
   a. Title I of the Health Insurance Portability and Accountability Act of 1997 (HIPAA)
   b. Title IX of the Medicare Prescription Drug, Improvement, and Modernization Act (MMA)
   c. Title XIX of the Social Security Acts
   d. Title XVIII of the Social Security Acts

2. In 2007, which standard claim form will be submitted by health care institutions to payers for inpatient and outpatient services?
   a. CMS-450
   b. CMS-1500
   c. UB-04
   d. UB-92

3. Which government-sponsored program provides health care services to members of the uniformed services and their families?
   a. CHAMPVA
   b. Military Health System (MHS)
   c. PACE
   d. SCHIP

4. The direct contract model, the individual practice association, and the network model are examples of which type of managed care plan?
   a. closed-panel health maintenance organization
   b. integrated delivery system
   c. open-panel health maintenance organization
   d. triple option plan

5. Which is true of a consumer-directed health plan (CDHP)?
   a. Individuals assume higher cost-sharing expenses after the designated amount has been expended.
   b. Individuals have less freedom in spending health care dollars up to a designated amount.
   c. Individuals receive full coverage for all of their in-network care.
   d. It does not provide individuals with an incentive to control costs of health benefits and health care.

6. Which models are included in the integrated delivery system managed care plan?
   a. flexible spending account, health care reimbursement account, and health reimbursement arrangement
   b. open-panel and closed-panel health maintenance organizations
   c. physician-hospital organization, management service organization, and group practice without walls
   d. point-of-service plan and preferred provider plan

7. Antoinette is preparing to transfer information regarding an inpatient encounter into the hospital's computerized patient accounting system. She uses a document that contains a list of procedures, services, and supplies along with the department code, service code and description, and revenue codes and charges. The document she is referencing is called a(n)
   a. chargemaster.
   b. CMS-1500.
   c. encounter form.
   d. UB-92.

8. The services that Allen received during his inpatient hospitalization resulted in expenses that were much higher than those of other cases in the same diagnosis-related group (DRG). Because these services qualified for additional reimbursement, his case was categorized as a(n):
   a. cost outlier.
   b. day outlier.
   c. exclusion.
   d. indemnification.

9. Which legislation resulted in the implementation of the skilled nursing facility prospective payment system (SNFPPS)?
   a. Balanced Budget Act of 1997
   b. Balanced Budget Refinement Act of 1999
   c. Omnibus Consolidated and Emergency Supplemental Appropriations Act of 1999
   d. Tax Equity and Fiscal Responsibility Act of 1983

10. Leon had some lab work completed as an outpatient on Wednesday in preparation for an inpatient procedure that was to be performed on Thursday. Under the prospective payment system, the lab work will be covered by the diagnosis-related group (DRG) payment. What is the name of the rule that ensures this?
    a. IPPS 3-day payment window
    b. IRF PPS 1-day payment window
    c. LTCH PPS 1-day payment window
    d. OPPS 3-day payment window

11. Which were implemented as a result of the Balanced Budget Act of 1997?
    a. IPPS, HH PPS, and OPPS
    b. IPPS, SNF PPS, and LTCH PPS
    c. OPPS, IRF PPS, and LTCH PPS
    d. SNF PPS, OPPS, and IRF PPS

12. Critical pathways:
    a. are standard procedures developed by hospitals to facilitate management and delivery of care.
    b. focus on the services provided by an individual discipline.
    c. provide opportunities for collaborative practice and team approaches between disciplines.
    d. rarely target clinical services that are high in volume and resource use.

13. The difference between fraud and abuse is the:
    a. concern that fraud involves much greater losses than abuse.
    b. fact that fraud is unintentional while abuse is deliberate.
    c. intent of the individual who committed the act.
    d. resultant damage or loss from fraudulent acts.

14. A provider bills Medicare for services that were never provided to a patient, is found guilty of fraud, and is ordered to pay a fine of $10,000 plus damages. Which of the following supports this decision?
    a. Civil Monetary Penalties Act
    b. Federal Claims Collection Act
    c. Payment Error and Prevention Program (PEPP)
    d. Stark I

15. A claim is submitted that contains codes for reconstruction of a female urethra (53430) and reconstruction of a male urethra (53410). The claim will be denied because 53430 and 53410 are _____ codes.
    a. component
    b. comprehensive
    c. manifestation
    d. mutually exclusive

16. Which is not applicable where there is an indication of fraud?
    a. Civil Monetary Penalties Act
    b. False Claims Act (FCA)
    c. federal antikickback statute
    d. Federal Claims Collection Act of 1966

17. Which resulted from the discovery that some health care organizations were billing Medicare Part B for services that were already paid under Part A?
    a. antikickback statute
    b. Payment Error and Prevention Program (PEPP)
    c. Physicians at Teaching Hospitals (PATH) initiative
    d. safe harbor regulations

18. Which statement describes a characteristic of a flat file?
    a. A flat file consists of a series of variable-length records.
    b. A flat file is not accepted by Medicare administrative contractors for claims submission.
    c. A flat file is used to bill institutional, professional, dental, and drug claims.
    d. Medicare administrative contractors send electronic remittance advices in the flat file format.

19. Which is not considered electronic data interchange (EDI)?
    a. ANSI ASC X12 837
    b. computer-generated paper claim
    c. flat file
    d. National Standard Format (NSF)

20. Locking the record storage areas at all times and limiting access to authorized users is an example of a:
    a. clinical protocol.
    b. confidentiality standard.
    c. privacy measure.
    d. security provision.

ANSWER KEY TO EXAM: CHAPTER 1

1. c	8. a	15. c
2. a	9. d	16. b
3. b	10. c	17. a
4. a	11. c	18. d
5. a	12. b	19. d
6. a	13. a	20. d
7. b	14. a	

ANSWER KEY TO EXAM: CHAPTER 2

1. d	8. a	15. d
2. b	9. a	16. d
3. a	10. d	17. c
4. b	11. a	18. d
5. a	12. b	19. b
6. a	13. d	20. b
7. d	14. c	

ANSWER KEY TO EXAM: CHAPTER 3

1. a	8. d	15. c
2. a	9. c	16. a
3. c	10. b	17. c
4. c	11. b	18. b
5. d	12. b	19. c
6. c	13. a	20. c
7. d	14. a	

ANSWER KEY TO EXAM: CHAPTER 4

1. a	3. c	5. d
2. d	4. c	6. b

> **Note:**
>
> *The delivery of an oversized infant (635.51) requires assignment of fifth digit 1. The hematoma was a postdelivery complication (674.32), which means that fifth digit 2 is assigned.*

7. d	12. a	17. b
8. a	13. b	18. a
9. b	14. d	19. d
10. d	15. a	20. b
11. b	16. a	

Note:

Superficial injuries (e.g., abrasions or contusions) are not coded when associated with more severe injuries to the same site. Because there was a left leg laceration (891.0), leg contusions (924.5) are not coded.

ANSWER KEY TO EXAM: CHAPTER 5

1. d	8. c	15. a
2. c	9. c	16. a
3. c	10. d	17. a
4. d	11. a	18. d
5. c	12. d	19. c
6. b	13. b	20. b
7. a	14. d	

ANSWER KEY TO EXAM: CHAPTER 6

1. d	8. b	15. c
2. b	9. b	16. a
3. d	10. b	17. a
4. d	11. b	18. a
5. c	12. a	19. b
6. d	13. d	20. c
7. a	14. d	

ANSWER KEY TO EXAM: CHAPTER 7

1. a	8. a	15. d
2. a	9. a	16. d
3. c	10. a	17. c
4. c	11. a	18. d
5. b	12. c	19. c
6. c	13. c	20. b
7. a	14. b	

ANSWER KEY TO EXAM: CHAPTER 8

1. c	8. b	15. a
2. c	9. c	16. c
3. b	10. d	17. b
4. a	11. a	18. c
5. c	12. d	19. c
6. d	13. c	20. c
7. b	14. a	

ANSWER KEY TO EXAM: CHAPTER 9

1. d	8. d	15. b
2. a	9. d	16. b
3. c	10. c	17. c
4. d	11. c	18. a
5. d	12. d	19. c
6. d	13. d	20. c
7. b	14. c	

ANSWER KEY TO EXAM: CHAPTER 10

1. a	4. a	7. a
2. d	5. c	
3. c	6. b	

Note:

The formula for calculating the anesthesia fee is [code-specific base unit value + anesthesia time unit(s) + modifying unit(s)] × locality-specific anesthesia conversion factor. The code-specific base unit value is 5. Anesthesia services were provided for 45 minutes. Anesthesia time units are counted in 15 minute sections; so (45 ÷ 15) will give you the number of anesthesia time units, which is 3. The patient is healthy; so a physical status modifier of -P1 is assigned, which has a relative value of 1 (the modifying unit). Thus, (5 + 3 + 1) × $19.20 = $172.80.

8. a	11. c	14. b
9. d	12. b	15. d
10. c	13. b	

Note:

Morbid obesity is assigned physical status modifier -P3, while obesity would be assigned physical status modifier -P2.

16. c	18. a	20. c
17. b	19. c	

ANSWER KEY TO EXAM: CHAPTER 11

1. a	8. a	15. d
2. a	9. b	16. c
3. a	10. d	17. d
4. c	11. d	18. c
5. c	12. c	19. d
6. c	13. c	20. a
7. b	14. b	

ANSWER KEY TO EXAM: CHAPTER 12

1. b	8. d	15. d
2. c	9. b	16. b
3. d	10. c	17. c
4. a	11. d	18. c
5. c	12. b	19. c
6. b	13. a	20. c
7. b	14. c	

ANSWER KEY TO EXAM: CHAPTER 13

1. b	8. c	15. d
2. b	9. c	16. d
3. c	10. a	17. d
4. d	11. d	18. b
5. c	12. c	19. b
6. d	13. c	20. c
7. b	14. a	

ANSWER KEY TO EXAM: CHAPTER 14

1. b	8. b	15. a
2. c	9. d	16. d
3. d	10. c	17. a
4. b	11. b	18. a
5. b	12. c	19. b
6. d	13. a	20. d
7. d	14. c	

ANSWER KEY TO EXAM: CHAPTER 15

1. d	8. a	15. a
2. b	9. b	16. b
3. a	10. b	17. c
4. a	11. d	18. b
5. a	12. c	19. a
6. c	13. a	20. a
7. a	14. b	

ANSWER KEY TO EXAM: CHAPTER 16

1. c	8. d	15. b
2. a	9. a	16. c
3. a	10. c	17. a
4. c	11. c	18. d
5. b	12. b	19. b
6. a	13. b	20. b
7. b	14. b	

ANSWER KEY TO EXAM: CHAPTER 17

1. b	8. b	15. a
2. c	9. d	16. c
3. c	10. a	17. c
4. d	11. d	18. a
5. b	12. c	19. a
6. c	13. b	20. a
7. a	14. b	

ANSWER KEY TO EXAM: CHAPTER 18

1. c	8. c	15. b
2. b	9. d	16. d
3. d	10. b	17. d
4. d	11. d	18. c
5. a	12. c	19. c
6. d	13. a	20. b
7. b	14. a	

ANSWER KEY TO EXAM: CHAPTER 19

1. b	8. a	15. d
2. c	9. a	16. d
3. b	10. a	17. c
4. c	11. d	18. b
5. a	12. c	19. b
6. c	13. c	20. d
7. a	14. a	

Answer Keys to Workbook Assignments and Reviews

Chapter 1
Overview of Coding

ASSIGNMENT 1.1 – CAREER AS A CODER: INTERVIEW OF A CODING PROFESSIONAL

The student will submit in paragraph format (not Q&A) a two- to three-page word-processed interview of a coding professional. Each paragraph should contain a minimum of three sentences, and the student should write in complete sentences. The paper should contain no typographical or grammatical errors. The last paragraph of the paper should summarize what the student's reaction to the interview was and whether the student would be interested in having this professional's position (along with an explanation of why or why not). Also, the student should "predict the future" by writing about where he or she will be in ten years in terms of employment, family, and so on.

ASSIGNMENT 1.2 – PROFESSIONAL DISCUSSION FORUMS (LISTSERV)

The student will go to http://list.nih.gov and click on "What Is LISTERV?" to learn all about online discussion forums (listservs). The student will also select a professional discussion forum from Table 1-1 in the Workbook and follow its instructions to become a member. If this assignment is completed by the student outside of class, the instructor can require the student to submit a summary of the experience (or if teaching online, post a discussion).

ASSIGNMENT 1.3 – VALIDATING ACCURACY OF ICD CODES

(Adapted and reprinted with permission from the American Health Information Management Association. Copyright © 1983 by the American Health Information Association.)

1. Code V55.1 is missing. It should be reported as an other (additional) diagnosis. Correct codes to be reported include V10.04, V55.1, and 44.62.

2. Code 170.9 is incorrect because carcinoma of the bone is considered metastatic spread from an unknown primary; assign codes 198.5 and 199.1 instead of 170.9. Code V67.2 is incorrect because it would be reported for follow-up examination following chemotherapy; delete code V67.2. Code V58.11 (chemotherapy) is missing; add code V58.11.

3. Code 414.0 is missing its fifth digit. The diagnosis arteriosclerotic heart disease (ASHD) does not indicate the type of artery or graft; therefore, assign code 414.00. The coder should query the physician to ask what type of artery or graft is affected by the ASHD. Code 428.0 should be sequenced first as the principal diagnosis because ASHD is a chronic condition and would not result in inpatient hospitalization unless the patient received treatment, such as cardiac catheterization or coronary artery bypass graft surgery. Although congestive heart failure can be considered a chronic condition, it can result in acute inpatient hospitalization with the patient receiving nonsurgical treatment (e.g., respiratory therapy and medications). Correct codes to be reported include 428.0 and 414.00.

4. Code 041.4 should be reported as an other (additional) diagnosis. Correct codes to be reported include 599.0 and 041.4.

5. Never report code 650 with a complicated delivery code (e.g., 653.41). Delivery cases require reporting either code 650 or a complicated delivery code. Although code 653.41 is correctly reported for fetopelvic disproportion, code 660.11 should be assigned and reported first as the principal diagnosis for obstructed labor due to fetopelvic disproportion. Category code 653 contains the instruction to

"Code first any associated obstructed labor (660.1)." Outcome of delivery code V27.0 was not assigned, and it should be reported as an other (additional) diagnosis. Code 74.9 is missing its fourth digit; report 74.99 instead. Correct codes to be reported include 660.11, 653.41, V27.0, and 74.99.

ASSIGNMENT 1.4 – FACE VALIDITY OF DATA MANAGEMENT REPORTS

(Permission to reuse granted by the American Health Information Management Association.)

Section A

SERVICE	DISCHARGES	DEATHS	AUTOPSIES[1] #	AUTOPSIES[1] %	DISCHARGE DAYS	AVERAGE LOS[1]	CONSULTS	MEDICARE PATIENTS #	MEDICARE PATIENTS DAYS	PEDIATRIC PATIENTS #	PEDIATRIC PATIENTS DAYS
Medicine	725	40	8	(25%)	6,394	9	717	301	3104	0	0
General Surgery	280	10	3	30%	2,374	8	184	80	916	0	0
Cardiac Surgery	64	1	1	100%	1,039	16	35	26	431		0
Hand Surgery	26	0	0	0%	81	3	2	3	10	0	0
Neurosurgery	94	0	0	0%	1,429	15	39	12	266	4	39
Plastic Surgery	46	0	0	0%	319	7	19	7	97	0	0
Dental Surgery	25	0	0	0%	81	3	46	2	11	1	3
Dermatology	20	0	0	0%	289	14	56	6	83	0	0
Neurology	83	0	0	0%	776	9	183	24	284	0	0
Ophthalmology	87	0	0	0%	352	4	98	51	183	0	0
Orthopedics	216	2	0	0%	1,920	9	64	39	563	1	2
Otolaryngology	139	2	0	0%	705	5	87	16	168	4	7
ICU[2]	8	(1)	1	50%	128	16	1	0		8	127
Psychiatry	126	0	0	0%	3,624	29	97	7	317	1	8
Urology	108	1	1	100%	810	8	74	36	318	0	0
Gynecology	184	2	1	50%	853	5	55	11	93	0	0
Obstetrics	451	2	2	(0%)	2,099	5	14	0	0	1	2
SUBTOTAL	2682	62	17	27%	23,273	9	1,771	621	6,844	20	189
Newborn	310	0	0	0%	1,191	4	0	0	0	0	0
SCN[3]	38	4	1	25%	742	20	0	0	0	0	0
TOTAL	3030	66	18	27%	25,206	8	1,771	621	6,844	20	189

Section B

DISCHARGE DISPOSITION	# OF PATIENTS
Against medical Advice	15
Home	2,850
Home health care	10
Skilled nursing facility	37
Rehabilitation facility	39
Other hospital	13
Expired	(65)
TOTAL	3,030

Section C

RESULTS	# OF PATIENTS
Discharged alive	2,964
Not treated	0
Diagnosis only	0
Expired over 48 hours	54
Expired under 48 hours	12
TOTAL	(3,029)

Section D

TYPE OF DEATH	NUMBER OF DEATHS	AUTOPSIES #	AUTOPSIES %
Anesthesia	0	0	0%
Postoperative	8	2	25%
Medical examiner	4	3	75%
Stillbirths	4	3	75%
TOTAL	16	8	50%

[1]Round up mathematical calculations to the whole number (e.g., 8.82 is reported as 9).
[2]ICU is the abbreviation for intensive care unit, where patients who need constant monitoring receive care.
[3]SCN is the abbreviation for special care nursery, where premature infants, twins, triplets, and so on receive care.

Section A

Under the Deaths column of the table (Column 3, Row 14), the number of ICU deaths should be 2. Because the Autopsies # data column is accurate and the subtotal of deaths is 62, there is an incorrect data entry in a cell above the Total row. Upon review of the data in each row for Autopsies, # and %, the calculated ICU autopsies % is 50%, which means that there were 2 ICU deaths.

Under the Autopsies column of the table (Column 4, Row 2), the Autopsies % for the Medicine service should be 20%. The Autopsies % in the Medicine service data cell is incorrect because $(8 \div 40) \times 100 = 20\%$ (not 25%).

Under the Autopsies column of the table (Column 4, Row 18), the Autopsies % for the Obstetrics data cell should be 100%. The Autopsies % in the Obstetrics service data cell is incorrect because $(2 \div 2) \times 100 = 100\%$.

Section B

Under the Discharge Disposition section of the table (Column 2, Row 8, bottom left), the total expired should be 66. The Discharge Disposition, Expired, # of Patients data cell is incorrect because the total expired is correctly reported as 66 in the top portion of the table. (All data located in subtotal and total rows in the upper portion of the spreadsheet are correct.)

Section C

The Results, # of Patients, Total (Column 5, Row 9, bottom middle) should be 3,030. The Results, # of Patients, Total data cell is incorrect because 2,964 + 54 + 12 = 3,030, which also matches the total in the top portion of the table (Column 1) and the bottom portion of the table (Column 1).

REVIEW

Multiple Choice

1. b	8. d	15. b
2. c	9. d	16. b
3. b	10. b	17. d
4. d	11. a	18. a
5. b	12. a	19. d
6. a	13. c	20. b
7. d	14. b	

Chapter 2
Introduction to ICD-9-CM Coding

ASSIGNMENT 2.1 – ICD-9-CM INDEX TO DISEASES

1. Rheumatoid <u>arthritis</u>   <u>714.0</u>
2. Acute myocardial <u>infarction</u>   <u>410.90</u>
3. Pseudomonas <u>pneumonia</u>   <u>482.1</u>
4. Type 2 <u>diabetes</u> mellitus   <u>250.00</u>
5. Congestive heart <u>failure</u>   <u>428.0</u>
6. <u>Crush</u> injury of right index finger   <u>927.3</u>
7. Sickle cell <u>anemia</u> in crisis   <u>282.60</u>

> **Note:**
> The ICD index lists code 282.60. When reviewing the ICD Tabular List, you will assign a more specific code.

8. Comminuted <u>fracture</u> of lower end of tibia   <u>824.8</u>
9. Congenital cleft lip, incomplete, unilateral   <u>749.12</u>
10. <u>Hypertensive</u> heart disease or Hypertensive heart <u>disease</u>   <u>402.90</u>

ASSIGNMENT 2.2 – ICD-9-CM INDEX TO PROCEDURES

1. <u>Incision</u> and drainage (I&D) of skin abscess   <u>86.04</u>
2. Low <u>cesarean</u> section   <u>74.1</u>
3. Laparoscopic <u>cholecystectomy</u>   <u>51.23</u>
4. Transurethral laser-induced <u>prostatectomy</u> (TULIP)   <u>60.21</u>
5. Extracorporeal shock wave <u>lithotripsy</u> (ESWL) of kidney   <u>98.51</u>
6. Loop electrosurgical excision procedure (<u>LEEP</u>) of cervix   <u>67.32</u>

> **Note:**
> When a procedural statement includes an abbreviation or acronym (e.g., LEEP), be sure to look up the acronym in the Index to Procedures first. If you do not find a code for the abbreviation or acronym, locate the meaning of each letter in a medical dictionary to look up the procedure.

7. Colostomy <u>take-down</u>   <u>46.52</u>
8. Knee <u>arthroscopy</u>   <u>80.26</u>
9. Extracapsular cataract <u>extraction</u> (ECCE)   <u>13.59</u>
10. Abdominal <u>hysterectomy</u>   <u>68.49</u>

REVIEW

Multiple Choice

1. c	8. d	15. b
2. b	9. d	16. c
3. d	10. d	17. c
4. c	11. b	18. d
5. b	12. c	19. c
6. d	13. c	20. c
7. d	14. d	

Chapter 3
ICD-9-CM Coding Conventions

ASSIGNMENT 3.1 – APPLYING ICD-9-CM CODING CONVENTIONS

Format

1. 176.4	6. 732.8	11. 49.31
2. 285.1	7. 391.8	12. 58.31
3. 365.21	8. 300.11	13. 45.02
4. 772.2	9. 388.31	14. 09.41
5. 584.6	10. 088.81, 320.7	15. 15.4

Eponyms

16. 272.7	21. 690.8	26. 83.88
17. 767.6	22. 100.89	27. 05.29
18. 346.20	23. 275.4	28. 44.66
19. 422.91	24. 015.00, 720.81	29. 77.99
20. 114.0	25. 426.9	30. 52.7

NEC and NOS Abbreviations

31. 482.30	36. 374.82	41. 43.99
32. 724.4	37. 253.2	42. 09.59
33. 999.5	38. 296.90	43. 67.12
34. 098.2	39. 455.6	44. 83.09
35. 008.47	40. 514	45. 77.58

Punctuation and Symbols

46. 458.9	49. 284.01	52. 027.0
47. 730.20	50. 250.50, 362.01	
48. 242.00, 376.22	51. 250.40, 581.81	

> **Note:**
> Do not assign code 320.7 (meningitis) because there is no mention of that condition in the diagnostic statement.

53. 284.1	56. 08.42	59. 39.29
54. 486	57. 27.69, 29.4	60. 74.3
55. 472.0	58. 22.60	

207

Boxed Notes

61. 824.8
62. 813.32
63. 250.02
64. 807.05
65. 550.92

66. 915.3
67. 923.10
68. 715.95
69. 851.83
70. 303.00

71. 90.33
72. 81.06, 81.62
73. 55.69, 00.91
74. 90.49
75. 33.6, 39.61, 00.93

Tables

> **Note:**
>
> Items 76 to 80 are from the Hypertension Table, items 81 to 85 are from the Neoplasm Table, and items 86 to 90 are from the Table of Drugs and Chemicals.

76. 405.99, 592.0
77. 405.09, 255.0
78. 572.3
79. 402.10
80. 404.90

81. 162.5
82. 234.8
83. 197.8
84. 212.1
85. 237.9

86. 983.9, E980.6
87. 995.29, E935.4
88. 969.4, E950.3
89. 962.7, E858.0
90. 693.0, E930.0

Includes and Excludes Notes and Inclusion Terms

91. 277.39
92. 451.81
93. 013.30
94. 726.19
95. 098.41

96. 518.89
97. 736.79
98. 572.2
99. 362.70
100. 334.8, 356.1

101. 60.5
102. 57.71
103. 46.10
104. 43.19
105. 27.63

Other, Other Specified, and Unspecified Codes

> **Note:**
>
> Item 106 is an other and specified *diagnosis* code; items 107 to 109 and 114 are other specified *diagnosis* codes; items 110 to 111, 113, and 115 are unspecified *diagnosis* codes; and items 117 to 120 are other *procedure codes.*

106. 729.90
107. 576.8
108. 529.8
109. 459.89
110. 274.9

111. 006.9
112. 319
113. 241.9
114. 110.8
115. 259.9

116. 47.99
117. 36.99
118. 48.76
119. 85.89
120. 93.39

Etiology and Manifestation Rules

121. 282.62, 517.3
122. 536.41, 041.11
123. 710.0, 582.81
124. 590.10, 041.2
125. 421.0, 041.00

126. 334.0, 425.8
127. 006.8, 595.4
128. 117.5, 321.0
129. 608.0, 041.02
130. 202.30

131. 015.00, 737.43
132. 099.3, 711.13
133. 693.0, E930.0
134. 510.9, 041.81
135. 272.6

And

136. 474.11	141. 616.10	146. 681.00
137. 513.1	142. 627.1	147. 472.2
138. 523.33	143. 749.23	148. 427.42
139. 565.1	144. 776.4	149. 372.75
140. 592.1	145. 680.2	150. 344.02

Due to

151. 371.24	156. 482.81	161. 117.9, 484.7
152. 525.11	157. 103.2	162. 773.1
153. 708.2	158. 537.3	163. 364.04
154. 767.8	159. 598.1	164. 275.0
155. 032.89	160. 117.9	165. 130.2

With

166. 381.4	171. 398.0	176. 810.00
167. 583.7	172. 379.05	177. 466.19
168. 571.2	173. 287.39	178. 115.95
169. 780.60	174. 707.10, 785.4	179. 094.0
170. 276.4	175. 282.2	180. 487.1

See and *See Also*

181. 363.20	186. 386.48	191. 83.89
182. 424.90	187. 441.02	192. 93.08
183. 520.1	188. 944.00	193. 88.75
184. 526.4	189. 537.89	194. 99.43
185. 927.3	190. 566	195. 80.47

REVIEW

Multiple Choice

1. d	8. c	15. c
2. d	9. b	16. c
3. a	10. d	17. c
4. b	11. d	18. b
5. c	12. a	19. c
6. a	13. a	20. b
7. b	14. b	

Chapter 4
ICD-9-CM Coding Guidelines

ASSIGNMENT 4.1 – ICD-9-CM OFFICIAL GUIDELINES FOR CODING AND REPORTING

1. 380.10, 785.6

> **Note:**
>
> • Do not assign codes to hearing loss (symptom) or fever (sign), which are the result of otitis externa. (A symptom is a condition the patient complains about, such as sore throat, chest pain, or difficulty urinating. A sign is a condition that the provider can observe, such as throat erythema (redness), tight chest, or blood in the urine.
>
> • Do assign a code to the "swollen axillary lymph nodes" because "axillary" is the medical term for "of armpit," and it is likely that the patient has another problem that has to be worked up due to this sign.

2. 345.50   4. V10.87   6. 728.71
3. 250.00   5. 786.05

> **Note:**
>
> The description of code 728.71 in the tabular list includes "plantar fasciitis (traumatic)." This is a case of "trust the index" because the index entry for "fasciitis, plantar" is 728.71. When verifying in the tabular list, even though the description doesn't exactly match the diagnostic statement in the exercise, the index sent you to 728.71, so assign that code. (If there had been an "excludes" note in the tabular list directing you to another code, you would have followed that instructional note.)

7. 250.60, 357.2

> **Note:**
>
> Refer to main term "diabetes, diabetic" in the index, and locate subterm "neuropathy." The index entry includes two codes: 250.6 [357.2]. Verify code 250.6 in the tabular list to assign fifth digit 2 (type 2, not stated as uncontrolled), and sequence code 250.60 first. Code 357.2 is located in slanted brackets in the index; therefore, it is sequenced second because it is a manifestation of the diabetes. (A manifestation is a condition the patient develops as the result of already having another condition, such as diabetic cataracts. The index provides the clue to proper sequencing of codes because the manifestation code in slanted brackets is always sequenced second.)

8. 601.9   10. 483.1
9. 614.0, 614.1   11. 591, 600.90

Note:

It is acceptable to sequence code 591 first even though the diagnostic statement says "Hydronephrosis due to prostatic hyperplasia." When locating codes for "hydronephrosis" and "prostatic hyperplasia," notice that they are listed as separate entries in the index. Even though the "due to" phrase is documented in the diagnostic statement, ICD does not classify one as a manifestation of the other. Thus, code 591 can be sequenced first. (The ICD guideline about sequencing manifestation codes does not apply to this exercise because code 591 was not located in slanted brackets in the index.)

12. 438.12

Note:

CVA is the abbreviation for cerebrovascular accident.

13. 715.94, 906.4

Note:

The residual condition is sequenced first, followed by the code for late effect.

14. 411.1   15. 086.9, 321.3   16. 789.03

Note:

RLQ is the abbreviation for right lower quadrant.

17. 908.3   19. 277.02, 041.7
18. 034.0   20. 710.0, 583.81

Note:

SLE is the abbreviation for systemic lupus erythematosus.

ASSIGNMENT 4.2 – ICD-9-CM DISEASE CODING

Infectious and Parasitic Diseases

1. 091.0   5. 030.9   9. 072.2
2. 045.92   6. 034.1   10. 077.2
3. 008.67   7. 053.9
4. 005.1   8. 070.53

Neoplasms

11. 224.4   15. 228.04   19. 191.3
12. 211.3   16. 140.4   20. 183.0
13. 212.1   17. 208.00
14. 227.0   18. 202.50

Endocrine, Nutritional, Metabolic, Immunity

21. 246.8
22. 253.3
23. 267
24. 279.11
25. 270.1

Note:

PKU is the abbreviation for Phenylketonuria.

26. 256.31
27. 257.1
28. 251.3
29. 254.1
30. 255.12

Diseases of the Blood and Blood-Forming Organs

31. 285.0
32. 288.3
33. 283.10
34. 282.49
35. 281.1
36. 282.62, 517.3
37. 284.09
38. 286.2

Note:

PTA is the abbreviation for plasma thromboplastin.

39. 286.6
40 289.4

Mental Disorders

41. 291.3
42. 290.20
43. 295.50
44. 300.21
45. 304.00
46. 301.7
47. 307.46
48. 307.23
49. 306.4
50. 307.81

Diseases of the Nervous System and Sense Organs

51. 320.82
52. 331.11
53. 336.1
54. 362.18
55. 339.00
56. 361.12
57. 356.3
58. 355.5
59. 372.13
60. 354.3

Diseases of the Circulatory System

61. 397.0
62. 455.4
63. 443.0, 785.4
64. 446.5
65. 427.31, 427.32
66. 429.6
67. 429.2

Note:

ASCVD is the abbreviation for arteriosclerotic cardiovascular disease.

68. 428.0

> **Note:**
>
> Right heart failure is classified as congestive heart failure.

69. 412

> **Note:**
>
> MI is the abbreviation for myocardial infarction.

70. 401.1

Diseases of the Respiratory System

71. 474.10	75. 513.1	79. 478.26
72. 482.84	76. 518.84	80. 477.2
73. 478.6	77. 518.3	
74. 494.1	78. 491.0	

Diseases of the Digestive System

81. 523.40   82. 524.62

> **Note:**
>
> TMJ is the abbreviation for temporomandibular joint.

83. 530.5   84. 529.5   85. 536.41, 041.4

> **Note:**
>
> E. coli is the abbreviation for Escherichia coli.

86. 551.01	88. 579.1	90. 526.81
87. 572.1	89. 560.31	

Diseases of the Genitourinary System

91. 593.6	95. 593.0	99. 590.2
92. 600.10	96. 599.82	100. 595.1
93. 611.5	97. 588.0	
94. 599.5	98. 581.1	

Complications of Pregnancy, Childbirth, and the Puerperium

101. 666.04	105. 635.52	109. 651.01, V27.2
102. 669.32	106. 634.91	110. 644.21, V27.0
103. 630	107. 672.04	
104. 633.80	108. 674.14	

Diseases of the Skin and Subcutaneous Tissue

111. 690.11
112. 707.07
113. 706.8
114. 709.1
115. 701.4
116. 703.8
117. 705.1
118. 694.0
119. 692.77
120. 695.3

Diseases of the Musculoskeletal System and Connective Tissue

121. 729.30
122. 736.05
123. 737.20
124. 710.2
125. 712.95
126. 714.81
127. 727.42
128. 726.32
129. 726.90
130. 730.06

Congenital Anomalies

131. 743.33
132. 746.86

> **Note:**
>
> *AV is the abbreviation for atrioventricular.*

133. 744.23
134. 748.0
135. 749.14
136. 754.61
137. 755.31
138. 755.02
139. 758.2
140. 757.32

Certain Conditions Originating in the Perinatal Period

141. 760.71
142. 770.3
143. 767.2
144. 777.3
145. 779.82
146. 765.02, 765.23
147. 277.4, 774.31
148. 775.3
149. 779.3
150. 779.5

Symptoms, Signs, and Ill-Defined Conditions

151. 793.1
152. 790.4

> **Note:**
>
> *LDH is the abbreviation for lactic acid dehydrogenase.*

153. 789.59
154. 796.2
155. 794.4
156. 798.0

> **Note:**
>
> *SIDS is the abbreviation for sudden infant death syndrome.*

157. 797
158. 789.05
159. 790.93

> **Note:**
> *PSA is the abbreviation for prostate specific antigen.*

160. 790.1

Injury and Poisoning

161. 951.5   162. 807.4   163. 806.030

> **Note:**
> *C2 is the abbreviation for the second cervical vertebra.*

164. 811.02   167. 824.4   170. 803.03
165. 833.10   168. 826.1
166. 967.0, E980.1   169. 836.0

V Codes: Supplementary Classification of Factors Influencing Health Status and Contact with Health Services

171. V10.60   175. V58.64   179. V70.4
172. V17.2   176. V57.3   180. V77.6
173. V43.3   177. V65.3, 250.00
174. V53.32   178. V69.4

E Codes: Supplementary Classification of External Causes of Injury and Poisoning

> **Note:**
> *Refer to the Index to External Causes and Injuries to locate the E codes for statements in this assignment.*

181. E837.3   182. E870.6

> **Note:**
> *Refer to main term Misadventure in the Index to External Causes.*

183. E904.0   185. E960.0   187. E908.4
184. E968.7   186. E905.3   188. E876.0

> **Note:**
> *Refer to main term Misadventure in the Index to External Causes.*

189. 969.4, E853.2

> **Note:**
> *Refer to the Table of Drugs and Chemicals located after the Index to Diseases.*

190. E884.2

ASSIGNMENT 4.3 – ICD-9-CM PROCEDURE CODING

Procedures and Interventions, Not Elsewhere Classified

1. 00.22   2. 00.51

> **Note:**
>
> CRT-D is the abbreviation for cardiac resynchronization defibrillator.

3. 00.62, 99.10   4. 00.33

> **Note:**
>
> CAS is the abbreviation for computer assisted surgery.

5. 00.03   6. 00.12   7. 00.22

> **Note:**
>
> IVUS is the abbreviation for intravascular ultrasound.

8. 00.50

> **Note:**
>
> CRT-P is the abbreviation for cardiac resynchronization therapy pacemaker.

9. 00.53   10. 00.11

Operations on the Nervous System

11. 03.51	15. 03.53	19. 03.95
12. 04.81	16. 03.31	20. 01.11
13. 07.72	17. 01.59	
14. 04.01	18. 02.12	

Operations on the Endocrine System

21. 06.4	25. 06.95	29. 07.16
22. 07.11	26. 06.39	30. 07.54
23. 07.62	27. 07.52	
24. 07.44	28. 06.7	

Operations on the Eye

31. 08.42   32. 09.81

> **Note:**
>
> DCR is the abbreviation for dacryocystorhinostomy.

33. 11.22
34. 16.21
35. 16.72
36. 14.54
37. 11.60
38. 13.19
39. 08.21
40. 09.21

Operations on the Ear

41. 19.9
42. 20.61
43. 20.23
44. 18.71
45. 19.53
46. 20.42
47. 18.12
48. 18.79
49. 18.11
50. 20.31

Operations on the Nose, Mouth, and Pharynx

51. 21.21
52. 23.19
53. 27.0
54. 27.62
55. 28.3
56. 29.4
57. 21.03
58. 21.61
59. 22.11
60. 23.09

Operations on the Respiratory System

61. 31.92
62. 34.02
63. 34.83
64. 32.22
65. 33.22
66. 33.27
67. 34.24
68. 34.74
69. 33.99
70. 31.1

Operations on the Cardiovascular System

71. 35.91, 39.61
72. 35.81
73. 37.28
74. 39.51
75. 37.0
76. 35.23
77. 39.30
78. 38.94
79. 38.22
80. 35.34, 39.61

Operations on the Hemic and Lymphatic System

81. 41.43
82. 41.91
83. 40.23
84. 41.31
85. 41.5
86. 40.63
87. 40.54
88. 41.06
89. 41.33
90. 40.11

Operations on the Digestive System

91. 45.16

Note:

EGD is the abbreviation for esophagogastroduodenoscopy.

92. 45.73
93. 48.0
94. 49.73
95. 49.22
96. 51.11

> **Note:**
>
> ERC is the abbreviation for endoscopic retrograde cholangiography.

97. 51.23   98. 52.7

> **Note:**
>
> A radical pancreaticoduodenectomy is also known as a Whipple procedure.

99. 53.7   100. 54.59

Operations on the Urinary System

101. 55.21   105. 58.93   109. 55.23
102. 55.7   106. 58.0   110. 57.6
103. 57.32   107. 58.23
104. 56.85   108. 55.69, 00.92

Operations on the Male Genital Organs

111. 60.21

> **Note:**
>
> TULIP is the abbreviation for transurethral ultrasound-guided laser-induced prostatectomy.

112. 60.97

> **Note:**
>
> TUNA is the abbreviation for transurethral needle ablation of prostate.

113. 62.5   114. 60.96

> **Note:**
>
> TUMT is the abbreviation for transurethral microwave thermotherapy.

115. 60.11   117. 62.3   119. 63.73
116. 60.62   118. 61.91   120. 64.11

Operations on the Female Genital Organs

121. 65.24   122. 66.11   123. 68.79

> **Note:**
>
> Schauta operation is a radical vaginal hysterectomy.

124. 67.33	126. 70.22	128. 69.09
125. 66.8	127. 71.3	

Note:

D and C is the abbreviation for dilation and curettage.

129. 68.16   130. 68.31

Note:

LSH is the abbreviation for laparoscopic supracervical hysterectomy.

Obstetrical Procedures

131. 74.1	135. 73.6	139. 75.61
132. 75.38	136. 73.01	140. 75.1
133. 75.93	137. 72.71	
134. 72.4	138. 75.4	

Operations on the Musculoskeletal System

141. 77.47	144. 83.86	147. 81.54
142. 79.73	145. 77.23	
143. 81.11	146. 80.51	

Note:

TKR is the abbreviation for total knee replacement.

148. 81.43   149. 83.01   150. 83.14

Operations on the Integumentary System

151. 86.27   152. 86.07

Note:

VAD is the abbreviation for vascular access device.

153. 85.21	155. 86.24	157. 86.28
154. 85.94	156. 86.09	

Note:

Removing necrosed skin by washing is a type of nonexcisional skin debridement.

158. 86.25   159. 86.11   160. 86.64

Miscellaneous Diagnostic and Therapeutic Procedures

161. 89.19

> **Note:**
>
> *EEG is the abbreviation for electroencephalogram.*

162. 93.05

> **Note:**
>
> *ROM is the abbreviation for range of motion.*

163. 94.32	166. 99.07	169. 95.41
164. 95.03	167. 97.82	170. 96.14
165. 96.33	168. 97.23	

REVIEW

Multiple Choice

1. b	3. b	5. b
2. a	4. a	

> **Note:**
>
> *According to the AHA Coding Clinic for ICD-9-CM, "Secondary arthritis is confined to joints of one area, and is due to some external or internal injury or disease process."*

6. c	9. c	12. a
7. a	10. b	
8. a	11. d	

> **Note:**
>
> *If students ask why the procedure statement did not include "partial" or "total" cholecystectomy so a more specific code could be assigned, tell them that the intent of this review question was to determine whether students would carefully read the statement and code only to the extent documented (and not infer anything more in the statement). It is the application of the rule "If it wasn't documented, it wasn't done," which means not to code something that was not documented as having been performed. (Documenting a more specific code would be considered "overcoding.")*

13. d

> **Note:**
>
> *ORIF is the abbreviation for open reduction with internal fixation.*

14. c   16. c   17. a

15. c

> **Note:**
>
> *Do not assign code 99.10 because it is reported for hypodermic (below skin), intramuscular (within muscle), or intravenous (into vein) injections only.*

18. d   19. c   20. c

Chapter 5
ICD-9-CM Hospital Inpatient Coding

ASSIGNMENT 5.1 – PHYSICIAN QUERY PROCESS

1. c

> ### Note:
>
> - Alcohol use and gallstones are the most common causes of acute pancreatitis.
> - Do not assign codes to symptoms (e.g., midabdominal pain) when a definitive diagnosis is established. In this case, the patient was definitively diagnosed with acute pancreatitis and cholecystitis.
> - Do not assign a code to cholelithiasis because this condition was not evaluated during the admission; it will be evaluated on an outpatient basis.

2. c

> ### Note:
>
> - Do not assign codes to symptoms such as fatigue, shortness of breath, and chest pain when a definitive diagnosis has been established. In this case, the patient was diagnosed with congestive heart failure.
> - According to the AHA's *Coding Clinic for ICD-9-CM,* "Pleural effusion is commonly seen with congestive heart failure . . . pleural effusion documented only as an x-ray finding without the physician having made such a diagnosis should not be reported." In this case, generate a physician query to ask if the "pleural effusion" should be documented as the principal diagnosis (instead of congestive heart failure).

3. d

> ### Note:
>
> *Documentation indicates that the patient was administered insulin during the hospitalization, and the patient is discharged with a prescription for insulin. Although the patient receives insulin during the hospitalization and continues to receive insulin upon return to the nursing facility, a physician query should be generated to ask if the patient's diabetes is type I or II.*

4. c

> **Note:**
>
> Elevated blood urea nitrogen (BUN) and creatinine levels are indicative of possible renal disease, and the physician should be asked if a diagnosis should be added for coding purposes.

5. c

> **Note:**
>
> • The diagnosis of "ectopic pregnancy" does not include the type (e.g., interstitial). The physician should be asked to document the type so a specific code can be assigned.
> • Pelvic tenderness is a symptom of an ectopic pregnancy, and it is not assigned a code.

6. Upon review of this case, the coder should <u>query the physician to ask whether knee joint effusion should be assigned a code</u> because <u>that condition was addressed by a consultant but it is not listed as a final diagnosis.</u>

7. Upon review of this case, the coder should <u>assign codes to HIV and lymphadenopathy</u> because <u>the physical examination, diagnostic workup, and final diagnosis justify assigning those codes.</u>

8. Upon review of this case, the coder should <u>query the physician to ask that he or she document the patient's final diagnosis on the record</u> because <u>it is inappropriate to assign codes for conditions based on review of the record when the physician has not documented established diagnoses.</u>

9. Upon review of this case, the coder should <u>query the physician to ask that a diagnosis related to the prescribed antibiotics be documented (e.g., cystitis)</u> because <u>benign prostatic hypertrophy is not typically associated with an infection.</u>

> **Note:**
>
> Cystitis can be caused by urinary retention associated with benign prostatic hypertrophy (BPH). Antibiotic treatment would be indicated for cystitis, and the patient's symptom of painful urination also supports this diagnosis.

10. Upon review of this case, the coder should query the physician to confirm that "microscopic fractures at T1 and L5" should be coded. The physician should also be asked whether the patient has "possible osteoporosis" because fractures noted on x-ray were not confirmed as a diagnosis by the attending physician. (The diagnosis of compression fractures plus the performance of bone density testing indicates "possible osteoporosis.")

> **Note:**
>
> The age of the patient and the microscopic fractures provide clues that a physician query should be generated to ask if "possible osteoporosis" should be documented on the record. However, even if "possible osteoporosis" is documented, do not assign a code to this condition because it is a qualified diagnosis. (For an outpatient case, code signs and/or symptoms instead of qualified diagnoses.)

ASSIGNMENT 5.2 – SELECTING AND CODING PRINCIPAL DIAGNOSIS, OTHER (ADDITIONAL) DIAGNOSES, PRINCIPAL PROCEDURE, AND OTHER SIGNIFICANT PROCEDURES

> **Note:**
>
> *For this answer key, extra rows not used for a case were removed. Rows that include a heading (e.g., complications) remain (even if codes are not reported) so that a consistent format is provided.*

1.

	ICD-9-CM Code(s)
Principal Diagnosis:	162.3
Other (Additional) Diagnosis(es): (e.g., comorbidities, complications, and secondary diagnoses)	V15.82
Principal Procedure:	33.27
Other Significant Procedure(s):	

> **Note:**
>
> *The patient's symptoms of shortness of breath and chest discomfort are not assigned codes because a reason for these symptoms was documented (non-small cell lung carcinoma). The patient's history of tobacco use is assigned a code to reflect an increased risk factor for the non-small cell lung carcinoma disease. The patient's family history was not assigned codes because his complaints and the final diagnosis were related to body systems other than those associated with diabetes and hypertension.*

2.

	ICD-9-CM Code(s)
Principal Diagnosis:	V30.00
Other (Additional) Diagnosis(es): (e.g., comorbidities, complications, and secondary diagnoses)	755.01 755.02
Principal Procedure:	86.26
Other Significant Procedure(s):	

Note:

For newborn records, the principal diagnosis code always indicates newborn or new birth status. The condition of extra digits is called polydactyly; and because there is no combination code for polydactyly of fingers and toes, classify each separately.

3.

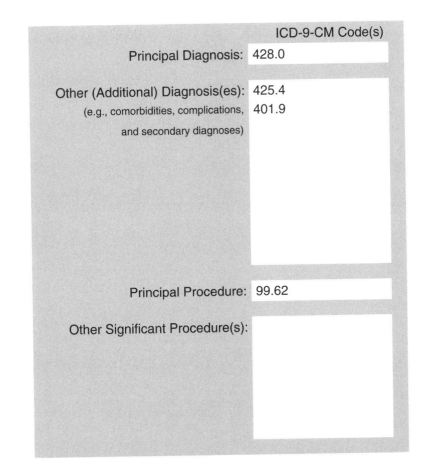

	ICD-9-CM Code(s)
Principal Diagnosis:	428.0
Other (Additional) Diagnosis(es): (e.g., comorbidities, complications, and secondary diagnoses)	425.4 401.9
Principal Procedure:	99.62
Other Significant Procedure(s):	

Note:

The signs and symptoms of respiratory distress, which include distended neck veins, systolic murmur, ventricular hypertrophy, and leg edema, are not assigned codes. All of these conditions are signs and symptoms of the patient's diagnoses: congestive heart failure and nonobstructive hypertrophic cardiomyopathy.

4.

	ICD-9-CM Code(s)
Principal Diagnosis:	V25.2
Other (Additional) Diagnosis(es): (e.g., comorbidities, complications, and secondary diagnoses)	997.1 427.89 E878.6 V08
Principal Procedure:	66.39
Other Significant Procedure(s):	

Note:

- Assign code 427.89 for postoperative complication of bradycardia an E code is also assigned (E878.6).
- Code V08 is assigned to indicate the patient's HIV-positive status.
- The ligation procedure code can be located by referring to main term *Sterilization* in the Index to Procedures. An alternative to locating the procedure code is to refer to main term *Ligation*.

5.

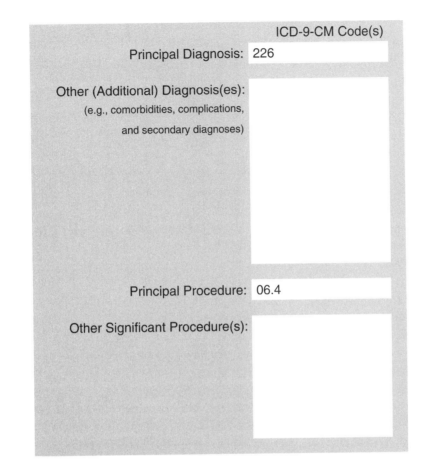

ICD-9-CM Code(s)

Principal Diagnosis: 226

Other (Additional) Diagnosis(es):
(e.g., comorbidities, complications,
and secondary diagnoses)

Principal Procedure: 06.4

Other Significant Procedure(s):

Note:

The coder should locate the diagnosis code in the Index to Diseases under main term Papilloma. *From there, the coder is directed to the Neoplasm Table,* benign, *and the specific site.*

6.

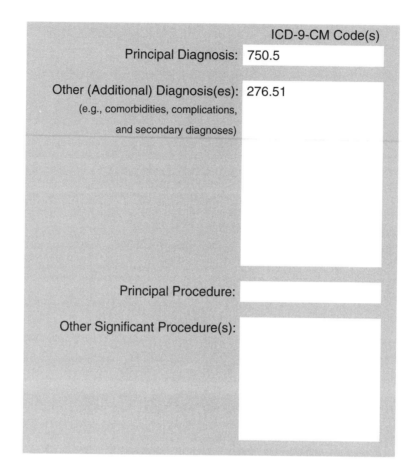

	ICD-9-CM Code(s)
Principal Diagnosis:	750.5
Other (Additional) Diagnosis(es): (e.g., comorbidities, complications, and secondary diagnoses)	276.51
Principal Procedure:	
Other Significant Procedure(s):	

Note:

In the Index to Diseases, refer to main term Stenosis, *subterm* pylorus (hypertrophic), *and 2nd qualifier* Infantile *to locate code 750.5. The patient in this case is 12 weeks old.*

7.

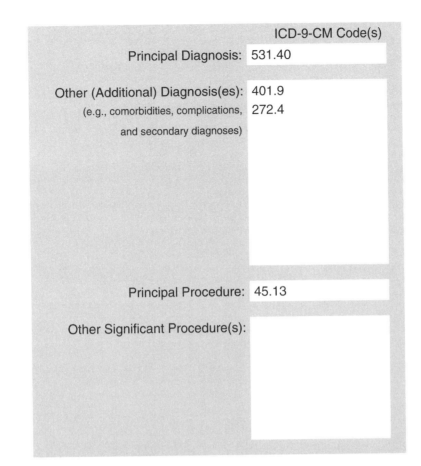

	ICD-9-CM Code(s)
Principal Diagnosis:	531.40
Other (Additional) Diagnosis(es): (e.g., comorbidities, complications, and secondary diagnoses)	401.9 272.4
Principal Procedure:	45.13
Other Significant Procedure(s):	

Note:

- The prepyloric peptic ulcer is described as "with acute hemorrhage," which means that combination code 531.40 is assigned. To assign the correct code, locate main term "ulcer," subterm "prepyloric," which directs you to "ulcer, gastric." Do not assign the code for "ulcer, peptic" because it states "site unspecified." In this case, the site is "prepyloric."

- The comorbidities of hypertension and hyperlipidemia are assigned codes because the patient's medication for these conditions was continued on this inpatient admission.

8.

	ICD-9-CM Code(s)
Principal Diagnosis:	188.0
Other (Additional) Diagnosis(es): (e.g., comorbidities, complications, and secondary diagnoses)	401.9 365.9 997.5 584.9 E878.6
Principal Procedure:	57.6
Other Significant Procedure(s):	57.6 45.52

Note:

- Assign code 584.9 for acute renal failure to indicate the specific type of postoperative complication; an E code is also assigned (E878.8).

- To assign code 57.87 for "partial cystectomy with enterocystoplasty, using part of the sigmoid colon," go to "reconstruction, bladder" in the procedure index. The patient underwent a reconstruction procedure because a bit of the colon was used to repair the bladder after the diseased portion of the bladder was removed.

- Code 57.87 contains a "code also" instruction to assign code 45.52 for resection of the colon (intestine). In this case, a portion of the sigmoid colon was used to repair the bladder after the partial cystectomy was performed.

9.

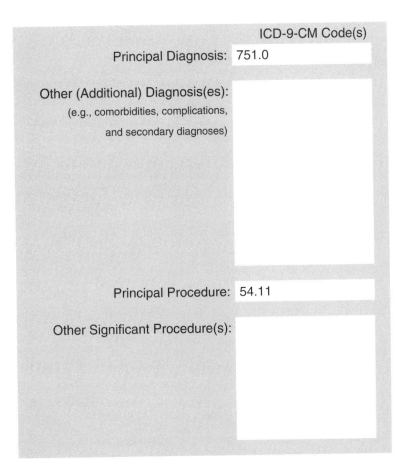

ICD-9-CM Code(s)

Principal Diagnosis: 751.0

Other (Additional) Diagnosis(es):
(e.g., comorbidities, complications,
and secondary diagnoses)

Principal Procedure: 54.11

Other Significant Procedure(s):

10.

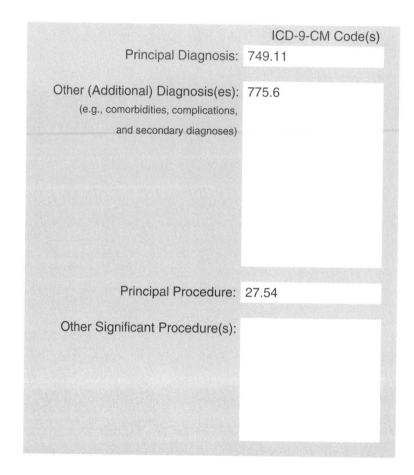

	ICD-9-CM Code(s)
Principal Diagnosis:	749.11
Other (Additional) Diagnosis(es): (e.g., comorbidities, complications, and secondary diagnoses)	775.6
Principal Procedure:	27.54
Other Significant Procedure(s):	

Note:

- A code from the V30 category is not assigned for this patient's discharge from Children's Hospital because the infant was not born during this admission.

- The condition of insulinoma was ruled out and is not coded. The code for hypoglycemia can be found by locating main term *Hypoglycemia* and the subterm *neonatal* in the ICD-9-CM index. There is no documentation that the infant's mother is a diabetic; therefore, do not assign code 775.0 to this case. Also, because the patient is an infant, do not assign code 251.2 for this case.

ASSIGNMENT 5.3 – CODING PRACTICE – HOSPITAL INPATIENT CASES

ICD-9-CM Chapter 1: Infectious and Parasitic Diseases

1. 084.6, 034.0

> **Note:**
>
> *Qualified diagnoses (e.g., probable exacerbation of malaria) are coded only on inpatient records. This means that back pain, low-grade fever, and chills are not coded because they are symptoms of malaria.*

2. 021.9

> **Note:**
>
> - Tularemia was the only diagnosis documented as treated during this hospitalization. Do not assign codes for the other (additional) diagnoses to past medical history diagnoses because they were not documented as treated. Do not assign codes to night sweats, fever, headache, poor appetite, dizziness, and weakness; they are symptoms of the tularemia.
> - Although the chest x-ray documented arteriosclerotic changes in the aorta, because the condition was not treated during this hospitalization, it is not coded.

ICD-9-CM Chapter 2: Neoplasms

3. 174.4, 196.3, M8010/3, 85.43

> **Note:**
>
> - Don't forget to assign morphology codes (e.g., M8010/3) to inpatient cancer cases.
> - Although the chest x-ray indicated some calcification of the mitral valve and dilation of the aorta, because there is no documentation that it was untreated, it is not coded.
> - Although lab results indicated a cholesterol level of 304, because there is no documentation that it was untreated, it is not coded.
> - Do not assign procedure code 85.21 to removal of breast tumor because that diagnostic procedure was followed by modified radical mastectomy, left during the same operative episode. Assign code 85.43 only for modified radical mastectomy, left.

4. 154.1, M8140/3, 48.50, 45.95

Note:

- Because there is no documentation that coronary artery disease and gastroesophageal reflux disease were treated, do not code them.
- To locate code 48.50, locate main term Resection and subterm abdominoendorectal in the ICD-9-CM Index to Procedures.
  - When verifying the code in the Tabular List of Procedures, don't forget to look for an instructional note. In this case, you are prompted to "code also any synchronous anastomosis other than end-to-end," which means that code 45.95 is also assigned.
  - The "includes" note below code 48.5 states "with synchronous colostomy." An ileostomy is a type of colostomy; it is a surgical opening created through the abdominal wall into the ileum so waste can be discharged from the body without going through the colon. Because the ileostomy was performed during the same operative episode as the lower abdominal resection, it is not separately coded.

ICD-9-CM Chapter 3: Endocrine, Nutritional, and Metabolic Diseases and Immunity Disorders

5. 250.02, 446.20, 447.6, V58.67, 38.21

Note:

- Pain in the hands is a symptom of collagen vascular disease and the qualified diagnosis (probable vasculitis of both hands) and is not coded.
- Code V58.67 classifies the long-term (current) use of insulin.
- Although hand x-rays indicated demineralization of bones, there was no treatment of this condition; therefore, it is not coded.

6. 276.8, E944.4, 462, 401.9, V58.67

Note:

- This patient sustained an adverse effect due to her diuretic medication; therefore, assign a code to the adverse effect (hypopotassemia) and to the drug causing the adverse effect (diuretic). (Use the Table of Drugs and Chemicals in the Index to Diseases to locate the E code.)
- Fever and chills are symptoms of acute pharyngitis; therefore, they are not coded.
- Hypertensive vascular disease is classified as hypertension, as indicated in the Index to Diseases, Hypertension Table.

ICD-9-CM Chapter 4: Diseases of the Blood and Blood-Forming Organs

7. 998.11, 287.31, E878.8, 27.52

Note:

- The case states that the hemorrhage is due to the idiopathic thrombocytopenic purpura. Since the condition is a postoperative complication, it is classified as such and assigned codes 998.11 and E878.8.
- Do not mistakenly assign code 86.59 for the mouth suture; code 27.52 is correct.

ICD-9-CM Chapter 5: Mental Disorders

8. 969.5, E853.9, 300.00

> **Note:**
>
> *An overdose is considered a poisoning. Refer to the Table of Drugs and Chemicals in the Index to Diseases to assign a code for the poisoning (overdose) and the external cause (tranquilizer tablets). The patient states that she was not trying to hurt herself; therefore, the E code is selected from the Accident column.*

ICD-9-CM Chapter 6: Diseases of the Nervous System and Sense Organs

9. 780.39, 437.0

> **Note:**
>
> *The possible lung tumor, as reported by the radiologist, was not treated; therefore, it is not coded.*

ICD-9-CM Chapter 7: Diseases of the Circulatory System

10. 437.7, 401.9

> **Note:**
>
> - The patient was evaluated and treated for transient global amnesia. She was also given medication for hypertension while hospitalized. Both conditions are coded.
> - The physician could be queried about the patient's elevated blood glucose level to determine if it is clinically significant and if it was treated.

11. 438.22, 438.11, 429.2, 250.00, 332.0, 412

> **Note:**
>
> - The patient sustained cerebrovascular accident (CVA) in the past and is treated during this admission for residuals of CVA (hemiplegia and aphasia), which are coded as late effects of the CVA. (Refer to main term *Late* in the Index to Diseases.)
> - Previous subendocardial myocardial infarction is coded as 412.
> - The patient's conditions of atherosclerotic cardiovascular_disease, Parkinson's, and adult-onset diabetes mellitus were treated during this admission, and they are coded.

12. 410.11, 496, 429.2, 412

> **Note:**
>
> *Code the status post myocardial infarction due to its clinical presentation during this admission and because this condition is significant to the patient's medical history.*

ICD-9-CM Chapter 8: Diseases of the Respiratory System

13. 482.31, 428.0, 707.03

> **Note:**
> - IV Ancef, chest physical therapy, and IPBB were done to treat pneumonia.
> - Lasix treated congestive heart failure.
> - Betadine and sugar compound treated the sacral decubitus.
> - Pleural effusion is a common symptom of congestive heart failure and is not coded unless specifically treated (e.g., a chest tube to drain the pleural effusion).

14. 493.22, 496

> **Note:**
> - Cough, shortness of breath, and difficulty breathing are symptoms of asthma; therefore, they are coded.
> - Chronic obstructive pulmonary disease is a chronic condition that was treated with Lasix and oxygen.

15. 518.81, 276.51, 414.00

> **Note:**
> - Shortness of breath is not coded because it is a symptom of acute respiratory failure.
> - In this case, peripheral cyanosis and hypotension are not coded because they are signs of acute respiratory failure and dehydration.
> - Atelectasis, noted on chest x-ray, is an abnormal finding that was not specifically treated during this admission; therefore, do not code it.

ICD-9-CM Chapter 9: Diseases of the Digestive System

16. 276.51, 263.9, 486, 599.0, 041.00, 331.0

> **Note:**
> - Code 263.9 is reported for malnutrition; based on information in the case, code 261 might be more appropriate; however, a physician query would need to be initiated to ask about assigning that code.
> - The patient's condition of Alzheimer's is coded due to its impact on her care during this admission and the fact that it was impacted by her dehydration and malnutrition.

17. 562.01, 45.25

> **Note:**
> - Diagnostic evaluation revealed jejunal diverticulitis.
> - A combination code is assigned for colonoscopy with biopsy.

ICD-9-CM Chapter 10: Diseases of the Genitourinary System

18. 591, V13.01, 55.51

> **Note:**
>
> - The conditions of TIA, hyperlipidemia, and hypertension are not coded because there is no documentation that they were treated on this admission.
> - The patient's nonfunctioning kidney is due to hydronephrosis. Nonfunctioning kidney is coded as V13.01.

ICD-9-CM Chapter 11: Complications of Pregnancy, Childbirth, and the Puerperium

19. 644.21, 642.51, V27.0, V25.2, 74.1, 66.32

> **Note:**
>
> - This patient presents at 34 weeks' gestation and delivers during this admission, which is classified as early delivery due to the number of weeks.
> - Severe pre-eclampsia is documented as treated with magnesium sulfate as seizure prophylaxis.
> - All delivery records must have a V code assigned to identify the outcome of delivery; in this case, a single liveborn infant.
> - The patient's wish for elective sterilization following delivery is coded, along with assignment of a procedure code.

20. 658.21, 664.01, V27.0, 75.69

> **Note:**
>
> - This patient underwent induction of labor after her membranes ruptured over 24 hours prior to delivery, which is classified as delayed delivery.
> - The patient also had a tear of her anterior perineum fourchette area during delivery. When an obstetrical patient undergoes episiotomy and sustains a perineal tear, code only the tear. (If the tear was repaired, a procedure code would also be reported.)
> - All delivery charts must have a V code to identify the outcome of the delivery; in this case, a single liveborn infant.

ICD-9-CM Chapter 12: Diseases of the Skin and Subcutaneous Tissue

21. 682.6, 278.01, 86.28

> **Note:**
>
> *The debridement of this patient's cellulitis was done via whirlpool, which is coded as a nonexcisional debridement.*

22. 873.51, E819.1, 86.59, 98.22

> **Note:**
>
> - Because glass (foreign body) was embedded in the laceration, in the ICD-9-CM Index to Diseases, locate *Wound, open, cheek, complicated.*
> - The fifth digit on E819.x reflects that this patient was a passenger in the motor vehicle.

ICD-9-CM Chapter 13: Diseases of the Musculoskeletal System and Connective Tissue

23. 535.00, 591, V13.01, 45.13

> **Note:**
>
> *Right upper quadrant abdominal pain is a symptom of gastritis; therefore, do not code it.*

24. 722.10, 846.0, 93.39

> **Note:**
>
> *There is no documentation of any injury in this case; therefore, do not assign an E code.*

ICD-9-CM Chapter 14: Congenital Anomalies

25. 753.14, 599.0, 041.4

> **Note:**
>
> - The patient was admitted for reevaluation of his polycystic kidney disease, which is reported as the principal diagnosis.
> - The urinary tract infection due to Escherichia coli found during admission is coded as an other diagnosis; two codes are required to report this condition.

ICD-9-CM Chapter 15: Certain Conditions Originating in the Perinatal Period

26. 558.9, 779.81

> **Note:**
>
> - Although the infant is just two weeks old, assign code 558.9 for gastroenteritis (because there is no code for this condition in Chapter 15, Certain Conditions Originating in the Perinatal Period). Lytren, Questran, and Nutramigen are antidiarrheal medications. Impending dehydration is not documented as having occurred and is not coded. Diarrhea is a symptom of gastroenteritis and is not coded. Urinary tract infection is not coded because the first culture proved to be contaminant.
> - The perinatal period begins at birth and lasts through the 28th day following birth, which means that code 779.81 is assigned for neonatal bradycardia.

ICD-9-CM Chapter 16: Symptoms, Signs, and Ill-Defined Conditions

27. 780.60, 278.01, 780.39

> **Note:**
> - The obesity resulted in difficult ambulation, and treatment was physical therapy.
> - The seizure disorder was treated with continuation of oral medications.

ICD-9-CM Chapter 17: Injury and Poisoning

28. 973.3, E858.4

> **Note:**
> - Fleet enema is a sodium phosphate intended to promote bowel elimination. Code 973.3 is found by locating main term *Sodium,* subterm *phosphate,* and the Poisoning column in the Table of Drugs and Chemicals, then referring to the Accidental column to locate the E code.
> - This patient did not show any signs or symptoms during this admission; therefore, no additional diagnosis codes are provided.

29. 964.0, 787.03, 787.91, E858.2, E849.0, 96.33, 96.39

> **Note:**
> - This case documents an accidental poisoning. Locate main term *Iron* in the Table of Drugs and Chemicals. Assign the code from the Poisoning column; then assign the E code from the Accidental column.
> - An E code is also assigned to indicate the place of occurrence (home).
> - Additional codes are assigned to describe manifestations, symptoms, or signs of the poisoning; in this case, codes for vomiting and diarrhea are assigned.

30. 807.01, 831.04, 486, 511.9, E819.1

> **Note:**
> *Velosef is an antibiotic used to treat the pneumonia. The shoulder dislocation and rib fracture were treated with analgesics. Qualified diagnoses (e.g., possible dislocation) are coded as if they were confirmed on inpatient records.*

Multiple Choice

1. d

> **Note:**
> *The Uniform Hospital Discharge Data Set (UHDDS) includes definitions of specific inpatient coding terms such as* principal diagnosis, other (additional) diagnoses, principal procedure, *and* significant procedure.

2. d

> **Note:**
>
> The insertion of a central line in this case is a significant procedure. The coronary artery bypass graft surgery is the principal procedure.

3. c

> **Note:**
>
> This case is an example of coding and reporting a symptom as principal diagnosis, followed by codes for comparing and contrasting diagnoses.

4. c

> **Note:**
>
> The principal diagnosis is the condition established after study to be the cause for admission. In this case, the principal diagnosis is the herniated lumbar disk.

5. a

> **Note:**
>
> Comorbidities are coexisting conditions, which means that the patient was diagnosed with them prior to hospital admission and those conditions were treated and/or medically managed during the hospitalization. They are, therefore, reported on the hospital claim as other (additional) diagnosis codes.

6. c

> **Note:**
>
> The principal diagnosis is the condition established after study to be the cause for admission. In this case, the nosebleeds and headaches are symptoms of hypertension.

7. d

> **Note:**
>
> In an inpatient setting, qualified diagnoses (e.g., possible) are coded as confirmed conditions.

8. b

> **Note:**
>
> This question is an example of an abnormal finding documented on an ancillary report. In this case, the atelectasis is not coded because the patient did not receive treatment or medical management of the condition. To code the atelectasis, the attending physician would need to have documented its clinical significance and/or treated the condition.

9. d

> **Note:**
>
> Both conditions (myocardial infarction and dilated cardiomyopathy) were present at admission, and both were treated equally. Per coding guidelines, either condition can be reported as the principal diagnosis.

10. c

> **Note:**
>
> Assign code V30.00 for term birth, single living infant; and report it as the principal diagnosis. Codes 650 and V27.0 are reported on the mother's claim, not the infant's; therefore, delete 650 and V27.0. Code 754.60 is correct for congenital talipes valgus. Correct codes to be reported include V30.00 and 754.60.

11. b

> **Note:**
>
> Per coding guidelines, the code for AIDS (042) is sequenced first, followed by the code for disseminated toxoplasmosis (130.8). The conditions of fever, headache, fatigue, and sore throat are not coded or reported because they are symptoms of the toxoplasmosis.

12. c

> **Note:**
>
> The final diagnosis of "likely fibromyalgia" is coded as if confirmed and reported as principal diagnosis. The symptoms of musculoskeletal pain of the neck, back, and shoulders are not coded or reported because these are common symptoms of fibromyalgia.

13. b

> **Note:**
>
> Adrenal hypofunction is also called Addison's disease. The admission diagnoses are symptoms of this disease, and they are not coded.

14. a

> **Note:**
>
> Acute pancreatitis is coded as 577.0.

15. c

> **Note:**
>
> The combination code for asthma with status asthmaticus is 493.91.

16. c

> **Note:**
>
> *Newborn dehydration is coded as 775.5.*

17. d

> **Note:**
>
> *Aortic value stenosis is not documented as rheumatic in origin; therefore, it is coded as 424.1. The aortic value replacement surgery with prosthesis procedure is coded as 35.22.*

18. c

> **Note:**
>
> *Although the fracture is closed, the treatment is open. Therefore, assign 824.8 and 79.36.*

19. b

> **Note:**
>
> *The postoperative bradycardia is classified as a complication of surgery. The principal diagnosis is carpal tunnel syndrome.*

20. d

> **Note:**
>
> *The maxillary sinusitis is documented as chronic (not acute). The Caldwell-Luc procedure involved removal of the lining of the maxillary sinus membrane.*

Chapter 6
ICD-9-CM Outpatient and Physician Office Coding

ASSIGNMENT 6.1 – PHYSICIAN QUERY PROCESS

1. d

> **Note:**
>
> *Even though the radiologist documented "frontal sinusitis" on the radiology report, the attending physician should be asked if she concurs that "frontal sinusitis" is the diagnosis that should be coded. Official coding guidelines state that abnormal findings (e.g., x-ray results) are not coded and reported unless the physician indicates their clinical significance. If the findings are outside the normal range and the physician has ordered other tests to evaluate the condition or prescribed treatment, it is appropriate to ask the physician whether the abnormal finding should be added. Also do not assign codes to the headache and facial pain because they are symptoms of the frontal sinusitis.*

2. a

> **Note:**
>
> *The patient's record clearly documents past history of type 2 diabetes mellitus and hypertension (HTN), which was also documented as medically managed during the visit. Type 2 diabetes mellitus justifies medical necessity for the blood glucose level, and HTN justifies medical necessity for the physician's writing a refilled prescription for Verelan.*

3. a

> **Note:**
>
> *This case is properly documented. A Colles' fracture involves the lower end of the radius with displacement of the distal fragment dorsally.*

4. b

> **Note:**
>
> *Assign a code for the toxic effect first (spider bite) and then the nature of the toxic effect (rash). The physician also has to be queried about whether the spider was venomous or not so the proper E code can be assigned, E905.1 versus E906.4.*

5. b

6. Upon review of this case, the coder should <u>query the physician as to whether a code for actinic keratosis should be assigned because official coding guidelines state that abnormal findings (e.g., pathology results) are not coded and reported unless the attending physician indicates their clinical significance.</u>

7. Upon review of this case, the coder should <u>assign a code for the skin tag, which was removed,</u> because <u>the skin tag was clearly documented in the case.</u>

8. Upon review of this case, the coder should <u>query the physician to ask whether symptoms of fatigue, blurred vision, and weight gain should be assigned codes because the diagnoses of hypertension and osteoarthritis do not account for the symptoms documented for this case. (NOTE: Do not assign a code to the osteoarthritis because it was not medically managed during this encounter.)</u>

9. Upon review of this case, the coder should <u>query the physician to verify that codes should be assigned to symptoms of flank pain, abdominal pain, and dysuria</u> because <u>although no diagnosis is documented, the ED physician may have established a definitive diagnosis based on examination and the results of ancillary tests.</u>

10. Upon review of this case, the coder should <u>query the physician</u> because <u>the type of burn (first-, second- or third-degree) is not documented. Due to documented blistering, the physician should be asked whether it would be appropriate to document for second-degree burns so a more specific code can be assigned.</u>

ASSIGNMENT 6.2 – DIAGNOSTIC CODING AND REPORTING GUIDELINES FOR OUTPATIENT SERVICES – HOSPITAL-BASED AND PHYSICIAN OFFICE

1. 463   2. 786.50

3. 466.0, 401.9, V16.1

> **Note:**
>
> *HTN is the abbreviation for hypertension. When acute and chronic conditions are treated during the same encounter, report the acute condition code first. In this case, report acute bronchitis code first.*

4. 214.1

> **Note:**
>
> *The abbreviation for diagnosis is dx.*

5. 493.92   6. V72.31, V76.47

> **Note:**
>
> *GYN is the abbreviation for gynecological. Pap is the abbreviation for Papanicolaou cervical smear.*

7. 881.00, 924.8

> **Note:**
>
> *The abbreviation for rule out is r/o. "Rule out" conditions are qualified diagnosis and are not assigned codes for outpatient care.*

8. V22.0   9. 592.0

> **Note:**
>
> *Do not report code 599.70 (hematuria), which is a sign of renal calculi.*

10. V57.21, V12.59

> **Note:**
>
> *The abbreviation for status post is s/p. CVA is the abbreviation for cerebrovascular accident.*

11. V382.9, 784.1, 228.01

> **Note:**
>
> *OM is the abbreviation for otitis media. The abbreviation for rule out is r/o. Hemangioma is a benign tumor.*

12. 780.79, 139.8

> **Note:**
>
> *EBV is the abbreviation for Epstein-Barr virus.*

13. 003.0   14. 428.0

> **Note:**
>
> CHF is the abbreviation for congestive heart failure.

15. 790.21

> **Note:**
>
> Generate a physician query for this case because, although a blood glucose lab value of over 126 mg/dl on at least two occasions confirms diabetes mellitus (American Diabetes Association guidelines), abnormal findings are not coded and reported unless the physician documents a diagnosis (e.g., diabetes mellitus).

16. 530.81

> **Note:**
>
> GERD is the abbreviation for gastroesophageal reflux disease.

17. 477.9
18. 577.0, 681.00, 785.0
19. 711.06, 041.5
20. 017.90, 420.0

ASSIGNMENT 6.3 – ICD-9-CM CODING GUIDELINES FOR OUTPATIENT DIAGNOSTIC TESTS

1. 715.97

> **Note:**
>
> DJD is the abbreviation for degenerative joint disease.

2. 369.8   3. V74.2, V01.89

> **Note:**
>
> "No bacterium found" in the diagnostic statement indicates that the patient underwent testing for Hansen's disease (V74.2).

4. 620.2, 796.2

> **Note:**
>
> Assign 796.2 for "BP reading 175/90." Another option is to generate a physician query to ask if a diagnosis should be documented for "BP reading 175/90."

5. 042, 136.3

> **Note:**
>
> *HIV is the abbreviation for human immunodeficiency virus.*

6. 599.70   7. 218.9   8. 253.5

> **Note:**
>
> *All of the symptoms and signs in this case are included in the diagnosis, diabetes insipidus. Therefore, do not code them separately.*

9. 255.0

> **Note:**
>
> - The signs and lab values in this case are included in the diagnosis, Cushing's syndrome. Therefore, do not code them separately.
> - Lab tests often include determining cortisol levels in blood. Cortisol is a corticosteroid hormone produced by the adrenal cortex (of the adrenal gland).

10. 442.81, 351.0   12. 836.0   14. 173.3
11. V76.11, V16.3   13. V72.83, 401.9

> **Note:**
>
> *BCC is the abbreviation for basal cell carcinoma.*

15. 959.01   17. 286.0, 356.9   18. 728.2, 728.87
16. 860.0, 807.01

> **Note:**
>
> *ALS is the abbreviation for amyotrophic lateral sclerosis, also called Lou Gehrig's disease.*

19. 422.90

> **Note:**
>
> *ECG is the abbreviation for electrocardiogram.*

20. 845.00

ASSIGNMENT 6.4 – SELECTING THE FIRST-LISTED DIAGNOSIS AND LINKING DIAGNOSES WITH PROCEDURES/SERVICES FOR MEDICAL NECESSITY

Selecting the First-Listed Diagnosis

1. Pain, left knee
2. Gastroesophageal reflux disease
3. Hypertension
4. Sore throat
5. Lipoma

Linking Diagnoses with Procedures/Services for Medical Necessity

6. e	10. g	14. h
7. b	11. i	15. d
8. a	12. j	
9. c	13. f	

ASSIGNMENT 6.5 – CODING PRACTICE

Ambulatory Surgery Center (ASC)

1. 246.1   2. 550.90, 752.51

> **Note:**
>
> Code 550.90 is assigned for right inguinal hernia because there is no documentation that the hernia is recurrent.

3. 550.90, 214.4   4. 574.31   5. 608.1

Chiropractic Office

6. 353.0

> **Note:**
>
> The patient's complaints of neck and shoulder pain are not assigned ICD codes because they are symptoms of thoracic outlet syndrome.

7. 724.3

> **Note:**
>
> The patient's complaint of gluteal pain with radiation is not assigned a code because it is a symptom of sciatica.

8. 724.4

> **Note:**
>
> The patient's complaint of low back pain is not assigned a code because it is a symptom of lumbar facet syndrome.

9. 729.1

> **Note:**
>
> - The patient's complaints of neck and back pain are not assigned codes because they are symptoms of myositis and myalgia.
> - When locating main terms *Myositis* and *Myalgia* in the ICD-9-CM index, notice that both are coded as 729.1. Report this code just once.

10. 847.0, 839.00

> **Note:**
>
> - When main term *Strain* is located in the ICD-9-CM index, the coder is referred to *sprain*.
> - When main term *Subluxation* is located in the ICD-9-CM index, the coder is referred to *dislocation*.
> - The patient's complaints of neck pain and muscle spasms are not assigned codes because they are symptoms of cervical sprain and cervical subluxation.

Hospital Emergency Department

11. 530.3   12. 709.00

> **Note:**
>
> - Locate code 709.00 by referring to ICD-9-CM Index to Diseases main term *Lesion* and subterm *pigmented (skin)*.

13. 883.1

> **Note:**
>
> The patient sustained an open wound to his finger when some PVC pipe entered the finger. The open wound then became infected. Infected open wounds are coded by going to main term Wound, subterm finger, and 2nd qualifier complicated to assign code 883.1 to this case. Do not assign code 958.3 (wound infection) to this case.

14. 729.5

> **Note:**
>
> In the ambulatory setting, the statement, sprain of right great toe versus early gout is not coded as a confirmed condition. The patient's symptoms are coded.

15. 780.2

Hospital Outpatient Department

16. V56.0, 250.41, 585.9, 583.81, 303.90

> **Note:**
>
> - The reason for care is dialysis treatment, for which code V56.0 is assigned.
> - The patient's end-stage renal disease (ESRD) is due to diabetes, and the ICD-9-CM index directs the coder to report ESRD as a secondary diagnosis for 250.xx (diabetes).
> - The patient has documented chronic alcoholism (303.9x); the patient is documented as being drunk during treatment, but the type of drunkenness is not stated. Therefore, assign code 303.90. Do not assign code 303.00, which classifies "acute alcoholic intoxication and unspecified drunkenness." The condition "acute alcoholic intoxication" does not mean that the patient has alcoholism. (For example, many people who were occasionally acutely intoxicated on alcohol during their youth were not later diagnosed with alcoholism.)

17. 784.0   18. 789.02, 790.6

> **Note:**
>
> *Qualified diagnoses (e.g., probable) are not coded for ambulatory or outpatient care. Instead, the patient's signs and symptoms are coded.*

19. 378.9   20. 780.60, 462

> **Note:**
>
> *Qualified diagnoses (e.g., probable) are not coded for ambulatory or outpatient care. Instead, the patient's signs and symptoms are coded.*

Hospital Same Day Surgery

21. 226, 401.9

> **Note:**
>
> *Hypertension is not documented by the physician as a postoperative complication. The documentation does not specify a type of hypertension. Thus, the coder cannot presume that the hypertension is malignant even though a blood pressure reading of 200/110 was documented. The hypertension is coded as unspecified.*

22. 585.9, 596.3, 600.00

> **Note:**
>
> *To locate the code for enlarged prostate, locate ICD-9-CM Index to Diseases main term* Enlargement, enlarged *and subterm* prostate *(600.00). The instructional note* "see also Hypertrophy" *next to main term* Enlargement, enlarged *also directs the coder to code 600.00 when main term* Hypertrophy, hypertrophic, *subterm* prostate *and 2nd qualifier* benign *are located.*

23. 474.10

> **Note:**
>
> Recurrent streptococcal sore throat is not a current condition, and it is not coded.

24. 836.0   25. 185

> **Note:**
>
> ICD-9-CM Index to Diseases main term Adenocarcinoma refers the coder to "Neoplasm, by site, malignant." This entry is located under the Malignant column in the Neoplasm Table.

Physician Office

26. 883.0   27. 381.4   28. 871.4

> **Note:**
>
> ICD-9-CM Index to Diseases main term Laceration and subterm cornea provides instruction directing the coder to subterm eyeball, where code 871.4 is located.

29. 490

> **Note:**
>
> Laryngitis and cough are not assigned codes because they are symptoms of bronchitis.

30. 843.9, 847.2

Stand-Alone Radiology Center

31. 722.0   32. 723.1   33. 721.0

> **Note:**
>
> ICD-9-CM Index to Diseases provides instruction to "see also Osteoarthrosis." Main term Osteoarthrosis and subterm spine provides instruction to "see also Spondylosis." Main term Spondylosis and subterm cervical lists code 721.0. If you mistakenly located code 715.98 in the index, the tabular list "excludes" note for that code directs you to codes 721.0–721.9.

34. 719.47

> **Note:**
>
> The patient does not have an ankle fracture or any other identifiable condition. Therefore, the symptom of ankle pain is coded.

35. 496

Stand-Alone Urgent Care Center

36. 346.90   37. 836.2

38. 413.1   39. 873.0   40. 284.1, 789.2

REVIEW

Multiple Choice

1. c	6. b	11. b
2. c	7. b	12. a
3. a	8. b	13. c
4. a	9. c	14. a
5. a	10. d	

15. b	17. a	19. b
16. c	18. a	20. d

Chapter 7
HCPCS Level II National Coding System

ASSIGNMENT 7.1 – HCPCS LEVEL II INDEX

1. Breast pump
2. Chemotherapy administration (OPPS)
3. Dialysate solution
4. External defibrillator electrode
5. Fracture orthosis
6. Liquid gas system
7. Oral antiemetic
8. Pneumatic nebulizer administration set
9. Pneumococcal vaccination administration
10. Wheelchair shock absorber

ASSIGNMENT 7.2 – HCPCS LEVEL II MODIFIERS

1. a	5. i	9. h
2. e	6. 8	10. b
3. d	7. c	
4. f	8. j	

ASSIGNMENT 7.3 – ASSIGNING HCPCS LEVEL II CODES

Transport Services Including Ambulance (A0000–A0999)

1. A0100	3. A0225	5. A0433
2. A0428	4. A0160	

Medical and Surgical Supplies (A4000–A8999)

6. A4349	8. A4367	10. A4556
7. A4338	9. A4458	

Administrative, Miscellaneous, and Investigational (A9000-A9999)

11. A9503	13. A9150	15. A9700
12. A9517	14. A9300	

Enteral and Parenteral Therapy (B4000–B9999)

16. B9004	18. B4103	20. B4102
17. B4082	19. B4176	

C Codes for Hospital OPPS (C1000–C9999)

21. C1722   23. C1785   25. C9723
22. C1880   24. C1750

Dental Codes (D0000-D9999)

26. D0274   27. D0475   28. D0330-EP

> **Note:**
>
> ESPDT refers to Medicaid's "early periodic screening diagnosis and treatment" program.

29. D1110   30. D3910

Durable Medical Equipment (E0100–E9999)

31. E0730   33. E0303   35. E0325
32. E0850   34. E1520

Procedures/Professional Services (Temporary) (G0000–G9999)

36. G0105   38. G0268   40. G0156 x 8
37. G0117   39. G0366

> **Note:**
>
> Code G0156 is reported for each 15 minutes of assistance.

Alcohol and/or Drug Abuse Treatment Services (H0001–H2037)

41. H2001   42. H0014

> **Note:**
>
> To locate the correct code, go to main term Alcohol in the HCPCS level II index and locate subterm abuse service. Then when verifying that code, review all codes in that section of the HCPCS level II tabular list to locate correct code H0014. (The HCPCS level II index is not as extensive as ICD-9-CM's index, and coders must review tabular listings to locate correct codes.)

43. H0030   44. H2014 × 2

> **Note:**
>
> Code H2014 is reported for each 15 minutes of training and development.

45. H0009

Drug Codes (J0000–J9999)

46. J0690   48. J0735   50. J3301, J3301
47. J0587   49. J2271

Temporary Durable Medical Equipment (K0000–K9999)

51. K0108
52. K0006
53. K0606
54. K0105
55. K0462

Orthotic Procedures (L0000–L4999)

56. L3001-LT
57. L1830
58. L3510
59. L2260
60. L1500

Prosthetic Procedures (L5000–L9999)

61. L8001
62. L8614
63. L6310
64. L6708
65. L8670

Medical Services (M0000-M0301)

66. M0301
67. M0076
68. M0300
69. M0075
70. M0064

Pathology and Laboratory Services (P0000–P9999)

71. P9057
72. P9010
73. P9022
74. P9043
75. P3000

Q Codes: Temporary Codes (Q0000–Q9999)

76. Q0113
77. Q4033
78. Q4049
79. Q0085
80. Q2004

Diagnostic Radiology Services (R0000–R5999)

81. R0076
82. R0070
83. R0075
84. R0070-UR
85. R0075-UN

Temporary National Codes (Non-Medicare) (S0000–S9999)

86. S9439
87. S2053
88. S0612
89. S3850
90. S9075

National T Codes Established for State Medicaid Agencies (T1000–T9999)

91. T1013

Note:

Code T1013 is reported for each 15 minutes of service.

92. T1027 × 2

Note:

Code T1027 is reported for each 15 minutes of training.

93. T2030
94. T1502-TE
95. T1000-TD × 2

Vision Services (V0000–V2999)

96. V2756
97. V2600
98. V2020
99. V2785
100. V2750 × 2

> **Note:**
>
> Code V2750 is reported for each lens that receives antireflective coating.

Hearing Services (V5000–V5999)

101. V5362
102. V5270
103. V5008
104. V5244
105. V5254

ASSIGNMENT 7.4 – HCPCS LEVEL II CODING CASE STUDIES

1. G0204-GH

> **Note:**
>
> Patient was seen for scheduled screening mammography. A suspicious lesion was found, and the patient underwent additional radiographic views. The patient's screening mammogram was converted to a diagnostic mammogram; therefore, add modifier -GH to the HCPCS code for diagnostic mammogram.

2. S0612, Q0091

> **Note:**
>
> Established patient presented for an annual gynecological examination, which included a screening annual Pap smear. In the HCPCS level II index, go to "Screening, gynecological, established patient" to locate the "annual gynecological examination" code. The CBC, thyroid panel, and complete metabolic panel are reported with codes from the Pathology and Laboratory section of CPT.

3. L8049-RT

> **Note:**
>
> Patient presents for modification of right ocular prosthesis device. Add modifier -RT to the HCPCS level II code to identify on which side of the body the prosthesis device is located.

4. S3841

> **Note:**
>
> This case documents two patients who are presenting for genetic testing for retinoblastoma. Report code S3841 on each patient's health insurance claim.

5. D2740

> **Note:**
>
> *This case documents the placement of a porcelain crown. There is no documentation that it was fused onto a metal; therefore, code D2740 is reported.*

REVIEW

Multiple Choice

1. c

> **Note:**
>
> *Ambulance origin and destination modifiers are located at the beginning of the Transportation Services Including Ambulance section of HCPCS level II.*
> - *Modifier -S refers to "scene of accident or acute event."*
> - *Modifier -H refers to "hospital."*

2. d

> **Note:**
>
> *IPPB is the abbreviation for intermittent positive pressure breathing device.*

3. b	7. c	11. b
4. b	8. b	12. a
5. a	9. c	13. b
6. b	10. d	14. d

> **Note:**
>
> *Imitrex is also known as sumatriptan succinate.*

15. c	17. b	19. c
16. d	18. d	20. c

> **Note:**
>
> *PSA is the abbreviation for prostate specific antigen.*

Chapter 8
Introduction to CPT Coding

ASSIGNMENT 8.1 – CPT INDEX

Identification of Main Term in CPT Index

1. Laparoscopic <u>jejunostomy</u>
2. Removal of a foreign body embedded in the conjunctival of the <u>eye</u>

> **Note:**
>
> *The main term can also be* Removal.

3. Suture of a <u>wound</u> of the kidney

> **Note:**
>
> *The main term can also be* Suture.

4. <u>Kasai</u> procedure
5. <u>Repair</u> of an inguinal <u>hernia</u>

> **Note:**
>
> *"Repair of an inguinal hernia" is indexed under main term* Repair *or main term* Hernia.

Identification of Procedure or Service as Main Term in CPT Index

6. Postpartum <u>dilation and curettage</u>
7. Ileum <u>endoscopy</u> via stoma
8. Clamp <u>circumcision</u> of newborn
9. <u>Arthrotomy</u> of toe, interphalangeal joint
10. <u>Gastrostomy</u> with vagotomy

Identification of Organ or Other Anatomic Site as Main Term in CPT Index

11. Repair of <u>diaphragm</u> laceration
12. Excision of <u>heel spur</u>
13. Excision of cyst of <u>pericardium</u>
14. <u>Pulmonary valve</u> replacement
15. Excision of epiphyseal bar of <u>radius</u>

Identification of Condition as Main Term in CPT Index

16. Toe <u>polydactyly</u> reconstruction

17. Repair of sliding inguinal <u>hernia</u>; patient is a 35-year-old male

18. Drainage of <u>cyst</u> of liver

19. Drainage of hip <u>hematoma</u>

20. Destruction of kidney <u>calculus</u>

> **Note:**
>
> *The main term can be "calculus," which is the condition of the kidney as specified in the area of the exercise (16 to 20). An alternative main term is "kidney," which is the anatomical location.*

Identification of Synonym as Main Term in CPT Index

21. <u>Albarran</u> test

22. <u>Binding</u> globulin, testosterone-estradiol

23. <u>Digital</u> slit-beam radiograph

24. <u>Energies</u>, electromagnetic

25. Urine test for <u>epinephrine</u>

Identification of Eponym as Main Term in CPT Index

26. <u>Blom-singer</u> prosthesis

27. <u>Waldius</u> procedure

28. <u>Dupuytren's</u> contracture

29. <u>Lee and White</u> test

30. <u>Ober-Yount</u> procedure

Identification of Abbreviation as Main Term in CPT Index

31. Manual sedimentation rate of <u>RBCs</u>

> **Note:**
>
> *RBCs is the abbreviation for red blood cells.*

32. <u>MRA</u> of the leg

> **Note:**
>
> *MRA is the abbreviation for magnetic resonance angiography.*

33. Urine <u>pH</u>

> **Note:**
>
> *The abbreviation for potential of hydrogen is pH, which is a measure of acidity and alkalinity.*

34. Standard <u>EEG</u>

> **Note:**
>
> *EEG is the abbreviation for electroencephalography.*

35. Complete <u>MRI</u> of the heart

> **Note:**
>
> *MRI is the abbreviation for magnetic resonance imaging.*

CPT Index Code Ranges

<u>75840–75842</u>   36. Adrenal <u>venography</u>

<u>61697–61708</u>   37. Intracranial artery aneurysm <u>repair</u>

> **Note:**
>
> *To locate this CPT code range, first index the word "repair," then "aneurysm," and finally "intracranial"; this will then identify the code range.*

<u>84702–84703</u>   38. Chorionic <u>gonadotropin</u>

<u>15300–15336</u>   39. Allograft <u>burns</u>

<u>33420–33422</u>   40. Mitral valve <u>valvotomy</u>

Use of the Directional Term *See* in the CPT Index

41. See Clotting Factor

42. See Fundoplasty, Esophagogastric

43. See Esophagomyotomy

44. See Chlamydia

45. See Antibody, Tetanus

ASSIGNMENT 8.2 – CPT APPENDICES

Appendix A

1. b	3. d	5. a
2. b	4. c	

Appendix B

6. b	8. c	10. c
7. b	9. d	

Appendix C

11. b	13. c	15. d
12. d	14. c	

> ## Note:
> CPT Appendix C code 99205 contains examples of cases that involve initial office or other outpatient consultation with patients who present with established diagnoses (made by another physician) or with an onset of symptoms that require a high level of service. In this case, the patient presents with recent onset of severe symptoms and the endocrinologist ordered a series of tests to evaluate the patient.

Appendix D

16. c	18. b	20. c
17. a	19. a	

Appendix E

21. a	23. b	25. a
22. d	24. c	

Appendix F

26. c	28. a	30. d
27. c	29. d	

Appendix G

31. b	32. c

> ## Note:
> EPS is the abbreviation for electrophysiological studies.

33. c	34. c	35. d

Appendix H

36. b	38. c	40. b
37. a	39. b	

Appendix I

41. b	43. b	45. a
42. c	44. b	

Appendix J

46. d	50. c	54. c
47. c	51. d	55. d
48. b	52. b	
49. c	53. b	

Appendix K

56. c   57. c

> **Note:**
>
> *Tdap is the abbreviation for tetanus, diphtheria Toxoids, and acellular pertussis vaccine.*

58. a

> **Note:**
>
> *AMA is the abbreviation for the American Medical Association.*

59. b   60. c

Appendix L

61. c   63. b   65. a
62. d   64. d

Appendix M

66. b   68. c   70. b
67. c   69. a

ASSIGNMENT 8.3 – CPT SYMBOLS

1. c   5. a   9. a
2. a   6. c   10. b
3. d   7. b
4. c   8. d

ASSIGNMENT 8.4 – CPT SECTIONS, SUBSECTIONS, CATEGORIES, AND SUBCATEGORIES

1. d   2. c

> **Note:**
>
> *DTP is the abbreviation for diphtheria, tetanus, and pertussis.*

3. b   6. b   9. d
4. a   7. b
5. b   8. b

> **Note:**
>
> *PET is the abbreviation for positron emission tomography, SPECT is the abbreviation for single photon emission computed tomography, and MRI is the abbreviation for magnetic resonance imaging. All of these are radiology scans.*

10. c

ASSIGNMENT 8.5 – CPT MODIFIERS

1. c	4. b	7. a
2. a	5. b	8. c
3. d	6. c	

> **Note:**
>
> *EGD is the abbreviation for esophagogastroduodenoscopy.*

9. b	14. a	19. c
10. a	15. d	20. b
11. c	16. d	
12. d	17. b	
13. c	18. b	

REVIEW

Multiple Choice

1. d	8. d	15. b
2. a	9. a	16. c
3. d	10. b	17. c
4. b	11. b	18. c
5. d	12. c	19. b
6. b	13. a	20. a
7. c	14. b	

Chapter 9
CPT Evaluation and Management

ASSIGNMENT 9.1 – LEVELS OF EVALUATION AND MANAGEMENT SERVICES

1. Subsequent
   Hospital Inpatient Services, Subsequent Hospital Care

2. New
   Office or Other Outpatient Services, New Patient

3. Not applicable (For emergency department services, no distinction is made between new and established patients.)
   Emergency Department Services

4. Established
   Preventive Medicine Services, Established Patient

5. New
   Nursing Facility Services

6. Detailed history

7. Expanded problem focused examination

8. Expanded problem focused history
   Problem focused examination

9. Expanded problem focused history
   Expanded problem focused examination
   Low complexity of medical decision making

10. Expanded problem focused history
    Expanded problem focused examination
    Straightforward complexity of medical decision making

ASSIGNMENT 9.2 – ASSIGNING EVALUATION AND MANAGEMENT CODES

	ICD Codes	CPT Codes
1.	782.1	99254

NOTE:
- Diagnosis code 782.1 (rash) is assigned because "rash due to allergy" is not classified in ICD.
- When a patient is seen at the request of another physician, consultation services are provided. Because this consultation took place during an inpatient admission, refer to codes 99251 to 99255.

	ICD Codes	CPT Codes
2.	948.32, 946.3, 250.00, 427.1, E890.3, E849.0	99284, 99291, 99292

NOTE:
- Although the patient was primarily treated for his burns, there is also documentation of treatment of ventricular tachycardia and diabetes. Therefore, ICD codes are assigned to each condition; and each justifies medical necessity for the evaluation and management and critical care services provided.
- The case does not include the burn site; therefore, code 948.32 is reported for the burn. In a health care facility, the coder should review the record to determine the burn site and/or initiate a physician query.
- The emergency department (ED) physician provided ED services to the patient, which is reported with code 99284. The physician documented 80 minutes of time administering critical care services to the patient; therefore, report codes 99291 and 99292.

	ICD Codes	CPT Codes
3.	780.79	99213

267

ICD Codes	CPT Codes
4. 493.90, 462, 783.0	99203

NOTE:

- Because sore throat and loss of appetite are unrelated to the asthma condition, all three conditions are assigned ICD codes. Each ICD code also justifies medical necessity for the evaluation and management services provided.
- Before assigning the CPT code, determine the level of history and examination and complexity of medical decision making. For a new patient office visit, three of three key components must be met or exceeded. The level of history for this case is detailed because the following were documented:
  - History of present illness that contained five elements (location, duration, severity, associated signs and symptoms, and modifying factors)
  - Complete review of systems
  - One element of the past/family/social history

Per the case, the level of examination is detailed and medical decision making was of moderate complexity.

ICD Codes	CPT Codes
5. 842.00, E888.9	99283

NOTE:

- Code the wrist sprain but not the wrist pain because it is a symptom of the sprain.
- Patients treated in the emergency department are not classified as new or established, and three of three key components must be met or exceeded to assign the appropriate code.
- Do not assign a CPT code for wrapping the sprained wrist with an Ace bandage because that service is included in the evaluation and management code.

ICD Codes	CPT Codes
6. 780.50, 331.0	99308

NOTE:

- "Difficulty sleeping" is located in the ICD index under main term *Sleep* and subterm *disturbance*.
- A code for Alzheimer disease is assigned to this case because the physician reviewed the patient's prescription medications to ensure that an adverse reaction would not occur when the patient was administered the newly prescribed sleep medication. Each ICD code justifies medical necessity for the evaluation and management services provided.
- Follow-up nursing facility care is called "subsequent nursing facility care" in CPT, and just two of three key components must be met or exceeded to assign the appropriate code.

ICD Codes	CPT Codes
7. 560.9	99221

NOTE:

- Assign an ICD code to the intestinal obstruction, but do not assign an ICD code to bone cancer because there is no documentation that it was treated.
- For initial hospital (inpatient) care, three of three key components must be met or exceeded to assign the appropriate code.

ICD Codes	CPT Codes
8. 728.87, 368.2	99243

NOTE:

- Assign ICD codes to muscle weakness and diplopia, both of which justify medical necessity for evaluation and management services.
- For office or other outpatient consultations, three of three key components must be met or exceeded to assign the appropriate

ICD Codes	CPT Codes
9. 729.1	99214

NOTE:

- Assign an ICD code to fibromyalgia, but not aching muscles because that is a symptom of fibromyalgia.
- An established patient office or other outpatient service requires that just two of three key components be met or exceeded to assign the appropriate code.

ICD Codes	CPT Codes
10. 466.0	99239

NOTE: Hospital discharge services include a final examination of the patient, discussion of the hospital stay with the patient and/or family, instructions for continuing care, preparation of discharge records (e.g., dictating the discharge summary), prescriptions, and referral forms. A key factor in selecting the appropriate code is the length of time the physician spent performing hospital discharge services.

ASSIGNMENT 9.3 – CODING PRACTICE

ICD Codes	CPT Codes
1. 401.9	99211
2. 959.01, E849.0	99219

NOTE:

- Refer to *injury, head* to assign the ICD code. Code E849.0 is reported to indicate the place of occurrence (home). The symptoms of confusion and disorientation are related to the head injury; therefore, do not assign ICD codes.
- CPT initial observation care codes require all three key components be met or exceeded to assign the appropriate code.

ICD Codes	CPT Codes
3. 453.40	99222, 93965

NOTE:
- Edema of the ankle and calf is a symptom of the suspected deep venous thrombosis and is not coded. Because this is an inpatient case, the suspected condition is coded as if confirmed.
- CPT initial hospital care codes require all three key components be met or exceeded to assign the appropriate code.
- The plethysmography procedure performed on this patient is classified in the CPT Medicine section.

ICD Codes	CPT Codes
4. 427.9	99244
5. 821.01	99283
6. 518.81	99291, 99292

NOTE:
- An ICD code is assigned to the acute respiratory arrest because that condition was treated by the respiratory care physician hospitalist. Do not assign ICD codes to chronic obstructive pulmonary disease with acute exacerbation, which is being treated by her attending physician during the inpatient stay. (A hospitalist is a staff physician employed by the hospital.)
- Code 99291 is reported for up to the first 74 minutes of critical care, and code 99292 is reported for each additional 30 minutes. (Code 99291 is reported just once on each date of service.) The patient in this case received a total of 105 minutes of critical care services. Therefore, report code 99291 for up to the first 74 minutes and code 99292 for the next 31 minutes.

ICD Codes	CPT Codes
7. 779.5, 765.07, 765.26	99295
8. 715.96	99325
9. 278.01	99349

NOTE: Do not report an ICD code for hypertension because it was not treated or medically managed during this visit.

ICD Codes	CPT Codes
10. V70.0, 401.9	99397, 99354

NOTE:
- ICD code V70.0 (annual examination) justifies medical necessity for the annual physical (CPT code 99397).
- ICD code 401.9 (hypertension) justifies medical necessity for prolonged services (CPT code 99354).
- Code 99354 is reported for up to the first 60 minutes of prolonged services provided by the physician. (A third-party payer might require an office or another outpatient service evaluation and management code to be reported instead of the prolonged services code.)

ICD Codes	CPT Codes
11. 079.4	99441
12. 414.00	99375
13. V20.0	99392
14. V30.01	99436
15. V70.3	99450

REVIEW

Multiple Choice

1. a   3. d   5. d

2. d   4. c

> **Note:**
>
> *This patient is at a high level of severity for presenting problem due to the intra-abdominal bleeding. If this medical condition is not addressed, the possibility for mortality is high due to blood loss.*

6. d	10. a	14. b
7. d	11. a	15. d
8. c	12. b	16. b
9. c	13. a	

Note:

The code range for this encounter is 99211 to 99215 since this is an established patient being seen in the physician's office. For established patient's, two out of three levels must be met or exceeded for a level to be assigned. An expanded problem focused exam and a MDM of moderate complexity met or exceeded the requirements for code 99213. (Code 99214 cannot be assigned because the physician did not document a detailed examination.)

17. c

Note:

All patients receiving ED E/M services are viewed as new patients; therefore, three out of three levels must be met or exceeded to assign a specific E/M code. Based on documentation, the ED physician exceeded the requirements for both examination and history; but code 99284 met the requirement of MDM for that level.

18. a

Note:

Initial inpatient consultations require that three out of three levels be met or exceeded. Based on the documentation, the consulting physician exceeded the requirement for the history and medical decision making component code 99253. The examination provided by the physician met the requirement of a detailed level, which is why code 99253 is assigned (and not a higher E/M, such as 99254).

19. d

Note:

For an established patient home visit, just two out of the three key components must be met or exceeded for a code to be assigned.

20. b

Note:

For an initial hospital care visit, all three key components must be met or exceeded.

Chapter 10
CPT Anesthesia

ASSIGNMENT 10.1 – DETERMINING ANESTHESIA SERVICE PAYMENTS

1. 01967-P2-AA   (Code and modifiers)
     5   (Base unit value)
     3   (Anesthesia time units; 45 ÷ f15 = 3)
     0   (Relative value)
     $16.52   (Conversation factor, Arkansas)
     $132.16   (Anesthesia service payment)

> **Note:**
>
> The formula is (5 + 3 + 0) × $16.52 = $132.16.

2. 01967-P2-AA, 01968-P2-AA, 99140   (Codes and modifiers)
     11   (Base unit value)

> **Note:**
>
> Reimbursement for multiple anesthesia services is based on the sum of base unit values because code 01968 is an add-on code. Anesthesia code 01967 has a base unit value of 5, and code 01968 has a base unit value of 6. Thus, the total base unit value is 11.

     5   (Anesthesia time units; 75 ÷ 15 = 5)

> **Note:**
>
> Modifier -P2 has a relative value of 0, and code 99140 has a relative value of 2. Total relative value is 2.

     2   (Relative value)
     $17.83   (Conversion factor, Arizona)
     $320.94   (Anesthesia service payment)

> **Note:**
>
> The formula is (11 + 5 + 2) × $17.83 = $320.94.

3. 00210-P5-AA, 99140   (Codes and modifiers)

    10   (Base unit value)

    4   (Anesthesia time units; 60 ÷ 15 = 4)

    5   (Relative value)

> **Note:**
>
> Physical status modifier -P5 is assigned a relative value of 3, and code 99140 is assigned a relative value of 2.

$17.04   (Conversion factor, Alabama)

$323.76   (Anesthesia service payment)

> **Note:**
>
> The formula is $(10 + 4 + 5) \times \$17.04 = \$323.76$.

ASSIGNMENT 10.2 – ANESTHESIA MODIFIERS

1. -G8   3. -AA   5. -P5

2. -QZ   4. -AD

> **Note:**
>
> If the ruptured spleen was not surgically repaired or removed, the patient would have died (e.g., from hemorrhaging).

6. -P4

> **Note:**
>
> ESRD is a severe systemic disease that is a constant threat to life (e.g., without dialysis or a kidney transplant, the patient would die). In this case the patient undergoes a procedure unrelated to the ESRD; but since the patient has ESRD, physical status modifier -P4 is added to the anesthesia code.

7. -P2

> **Note:**
>
> Chronic asthma is a mild systemic disease.

8. -74   9. -23   10. -59

ASSIGNMENT 10.3 – CODING PRACTICE

	ICD Codes	CPT Codes
1.	852.21	00214-P1-AA, 36620-59, 93503-59

NOTE: Do not assign ICD codes to vertigo or headaches, which are symptoms of the subdural hematoma.

2.	142.0, 401.9	00100-P2-QX

NOTE: Code 142.0 medically justifies anesthesia administration.

3.	925.2, E917.4	00326-P5-AA, 99140, 36620

NOTE:
• Do not assign ICD codes to the severe breathing problems or the patient's cold and sweaty condition, which was a result of the crushed larynx injury.
• Code 925.2 medically justifies anesthesia administration.

4.	198.89	00300-P4-QZ
5.	810.00, E885.2	00450-P1-AA

NOTE: Code 810.00 medically justifies anesthesia administration.

6.	198.5, 199.1	00470-P4-AA, 99100

NOTE:
• Do not assign ICD code 170.3 for bone cancer because unless stated as primary, bone cancer is classified as secondary (or metastatic) cancer.
• CD code 199.1 is reported for unknown primary cancer.

7.	996.01, 426.10, V45.01	00530-P4-AA, 99100

NOTE:
• Twiddler syndrome is a mechanical complication of a cardiac pacemaker in which the pacemaker leads inappropriately retract, resulting in inappropriate shocks to the heart muscle. (To assign the code for Twiddler syndrome, first locate the definition of the syndrome in your medical dictionary or on the Internet. Then go to ICD-9-CM Index to Diseases main term *Complication*, subterm *mechanical*, 2nd qualifier pacemaker, and 3rd qualifier *cardiac*. Verify code 996.01 in the tabular list.
• Do not assign ICD code 429.4, which classifies cardiac insufficiency that occurs after the immediate postoperative period. (It usually occurs years after initial implantation of the pacemaker.)
• Code 996.01 medically justifies anesthesia administration, and codes 426.10 and V45.01 justify assignment of physical status modifier -P4.

8.	150.9, 250.01	00500-P3-AA, 99100

NOTE:
• Code 150.9 medically justifies anesthesia administration, and code 250.01 justifies assignment of physical status modifier -P3.
• It is not necessary to assign ICD code V15.82 (history of tobacco abuse) for an anesthesia case because it does not impact selection of the physical status modifier. Also do not mistakenly assign code 305.1, which classifies current tobacco abuse. (If the patient was a current tobacco abuser, code 305.1 would be reported.)

9.	213.2	00620-P1-QX
10.	722.0, 250.00	00600-P2-AA

NOTE:
• Do not assign an ICD code to the upper back pain because it is a symptom of the displaced cervical intervertebral disk.
• Code 722.0 medically justifies anesthesia administration, and code 250.00 justifies assignment of physical status modifier -P2.

11.	571.5, 303.90	00796-P4-AA, 93503
12.	278.01, 401.9, 250.00, 272.0	00797-P3-AA

NOTE: Code 278.01 medically justifies anesthesia administration; and codes 401.9, 250.00, and 272.0 justify assignment of physical status modifier -P3.

13.	553.20, 413.9, 305.00	00830-P3-QZ

NOTE:
• Do not assign an ICD code to the lump in the lower abdominal area, which was due to an abdominal hernia.
• Code 553.20 medically justifies anesthesia administration, and codes 413.9 and 305.00 justify assignment of physical status modifier -P3.

14.	250.41, 585.6	00868-P4-AA, 36620-59, 93503-59

NOTE: Two ICD codes must be assigned to completely classify the diagnosis for this case.

15.	752.51	00924-P1-QZ, 99100

ICD Codes	CPT Codes
16. 997.99, 607.84, 042, V10.49	00938-P3-AA

NOTE:
- According to the AHA's *Coding Clinic for ICD-9-CM,* when impotence is the result of surgery performed to remove a malignancy, code 997.9 (Complications affecting other specified body systems, not elsewhere classified) is assigned, followed by code 607.84 (Impotence of organic origin) and code V10.49 (Personal history of malignant neoplasm, genital organs, other male genital organs).
- This case also indicates that the patient is HIV-infected, which is assigned ICD code 042.
- Code 997.99 medically justifies anesthesia administration, and codes 607.84, 042, and V10.46 justify assignment of physical status modifier -P3.

ICD Codes	CPT Codes
17. 808.8, E814.7	01120-P1-AA, 99140

NOTE: Code 808.8 medically justifies anesthesia administration.

ICD Codes	CPT Codes
18. 828.0, E819.7	01130-P1-AA, 99140

NOTE: Code 828.0 medically justifies anesthesia administration.

ICD Codes	CPT Codes
19. 454.0	01260-P3-AA
20. 820.8, E880.1	01220-P1-QZ, 99100

NOTE: Code 820.8 medically justifies anesthesia administration.

ICD Codes	CPT Codes
21. 719.46, 401.9	01382-P2-AA

NOTE: Code 719.46 medically justifies anesthesia administration, and code 401.9 justifies assignment of physical status modifier -P2.

ICD Codes	CPT Codes
22. 823.01, 250.00, E822.7	01392-P2-AA, 99100

NOTE: Code 823.01 medically justifies anesthesia administration, and code 250.00 justifies assignment of physical status modifier -P2.

ICD Codes	CPT Codes
23. 735.2	01480-P2-AA
24. 198.5	01470-P3-AA
25. 732.7	01630-P1-AA
26. 812.00, E885.9	01680-P1-AA

NOTE: Code 812.00 medically justifies anesthesia administration.

ICD Codes	CPT Codes
27. 927.11, 042, E882	01760-P4-QX

NOTE: Code 927.11 medically justifies anesthesia administration, and code 042 justifies assignment of physical status modifier -P3.

ICD Codes	CPT Codes
28. 733.20, 579.0, 272.0	01758-P2-AA

NOTE: Code 733.20 medically justifies anesthesia administration, and codes 579.0 and 272.0 justi assignment of physical status modifier -P2.

ICD Codes	CPT Codes
29. 813.81	01820-P1-AA
30. 814.00, E917.4	01820-P1-QX

NOTE: Code 814.00 medically justifies anesthesia administration.

ICD Codes	CPT Codes
31. 729.5	01916-P1-AA
32. 724.5, 250.00	01936-P2-QX

NOTE: Code 724.5 medically justifies anesthesia administration, and code 250.00 justifies assignment of physical status modifier -P2.

ICD Codes	CPT Codes
33. 948.00, 949.3, 305.1, 305.00	01951-P2-AA

NOTE: Codes 948.00 and 949.2 medically justify anesthesia administration, and codes 305.1 and 305.00 justify assignment of physical status modifier -P2.

ICD Codes	CPT Codes
34. 948.00, 945.20	01952-P1-QZ
35. 669.71, 042, V27.0	01963-P4-AA, 99140

NOTE: Code 669.71 medically justifies anesthesia administration, and code 042 justifies assignment of physical status modifier -P3.

ICD Codes	CPT Codes
36. 651.01, V27.2	01960-P1-QX

NOTE: Code 651.01 medically justifies anesthesia administration.

ICD Codes	CPT Codes
37. 651.11, V27.5	01967-P1-AA

NOTE: Code 651.11 medically justifies anesthesia administration.

	ICD Codes	CPT Codes
38.	V59.4	01990-P6-AA
39.	332.0	01992-P3-AA
40.	745.5	01996-P5-AA, 99140

REVIEW

Multiple Choice

1. d   2. d   3. a

> **Note:**
>
> The abbreviation for cesarean section is c-section.

4. b

> **Note:**
>
> ECG is the abbreviation for electrocardiogram. This procedure is also abbreviated as EKG.

5. b

> **Note:**
>
> CVAD is the abbreviation for central venous access device.

6. b   8. c   10. d
7. c   9. a

> **Note:**
>
> - ECT is the abbreviation for electroconvulsive therapy.
> - EMG is the abbreviation for electromyogram.
> - LP is the abbreviation for lumbar puncture.
> - MAC is the abbreviation for monitored anesthesia care.

11. c   15. d   19. d
12. a   16. b   20. a
13. b   17. a
14. b   18. c

Chapter 11
CPT Surgery I

ASSIGNMENT 11.1 – CODING PRACTICE

	ICD Codes	CPT Codes
1.	883.1	11760-FA

NOTE: The presence of a foreign object meets the criteria to assign a complicated wound code.

2.	216.5	11302

NOTE: To locate the ICD code, go to the Neoplasm Table in the alphabetic index and locate *skin, trunk, benign*.

3.	172.3	11644
4.	881.00, 881.02	12002

NOTE: Both wounds were repaired with simple closure, and they are grouped in code range 12001–12007. The wound sizes are added together to obtain a total wound size of 6.0 cm.

5.	680.6	10060

ASSIGNMENT 11.2 – CODING OPERATIVE REPORTS

	ICD Codes	CPT Codes
1.	569.49	11402

NOTE:
- To assign the ICD diagnosis code, locate subterm *anus* under main term *Cyst*. (There is no subterm *perianal* under main term *Cyst*.)
- A cyst is a type of benign lesion. Refer to the note located above CPT code 11400, which provides examples of terms that could be used when classifying benign lesions.

2.	686.1	11421-F6

NOTE: A granuloma is a type of benign lesion. Therefore, the CPT code range for its excision is 11400–11471.

3.	173.3	14040

NOTE: CPT codes for advancement flap procedures are located in the Adjacent Tissue Transfer subheading, and the code assigned reflects the recipient site of the flap (e.g., forehead). These codes include excision of the lesion, which means that a secondary procedure code for excision of the lesion is not assigned.

4.	707.04, 340	15958, 15738-51

NOTE: A decubitus ulcer is also called a pressure ulcer, and the procedure performed requires the assignment of two CPT codes. Code 15958 is assigned for excision of the ulcer, including ostectomy, and code 15738 is assigned for the muscle flap closure of the surgical defect.

5.	611.79	19355-50

NOTE: Although the description of code 19355 contains the term *nipples* (plural of *nipple*), modifier -50 is added to the code because the CMS/Medicare physician fee schedule assigns a value of 1 in the Bilateral Surgery column for this code. The CMS definition of value 1 for Bilateral Surgery (Modifier 50) states:

1 = 150% payment adjustment for bilateral procedures applies. If the code is billed with the bilateral modifier or is reported twice on the same day by any other means (e.g., with RT and LT modifiers, or with a 2 in the units field), base the payment for these codes when reported as bilateral procedures on the lower of: (a) the total actual charge for both sides or (b) 150% of the fee schedule amount for a single code. If the code is reported as a bilateral procedure and is reported with other procedure codes on the same day, apply the bilateral adjustment before applying any multiple procedure rules.

REVIEW

Multiple Choice

1. b

> **Note:**
>
> This patient's surgery requires assignment of one code for the excision of the 1.5 cm in diameter basal cell carcinoma lesion of the cheek and another code for the shaving of the 2.5 cm in diameter basal cell carcinoma lesion of the nose.

2. c	5. a	8. b
3. d	6. c	9. a
4. b	7. a	10. c

> **Note:**
>
> - The hand and foot wounds were repaired with an intermediate closure; the lengths of these wounds are combined based on the classification of the anatomic sites in CPT. The hand and foot wounds totaled 5.0 centimeter, and code 12042 is assigned.
> - Based on the classification of the anatomic sites in CPT, the lengths of the scalp and neck wounds can also be combined because both required simple repairs. The scalp and neck wounds totaled 4.0 centimeters, and code 12002 is assigned.

11. a	13. b	15. d
12. c	14. c	16. b

> **Note:**
>
> This type of lesion is classified as a benign lesion and is coded in the 11400 to 11471 range of CPT codes under the Integumentary System subsection.

17. c	19. b	20. b
18. a		

Chapter 12
CPT Surgery II

ASSIGNMENT 12.1 – CODING PRACTICE

	ICD Codes	CPT Codes
1.	835.00	27253
NOTE: This case documents a closed hip dislocation; however, treatment was open reduction of the dislocation.		
2.	491.9	31717
3.	754.30	27275
4.	813.43	25650
NOTE: The application of the cast is included in the code for the closed fracture treatment. Do not assign a separate code for the cast application.		
5.	511.9	32421
6.	874.02	31800
7.	464.00	31575
8.	802.0	21315
9.	729.71	26037
10.	578.0	31625, 31620

NOTE:
- For outpatient care, do not assign codes to diagnoses stated as "rule out." Assign codes to confirmed diagnoses or signs/symptoms when there is no confirmed diagnosis.
- Do not add modifier -51 to code 31620, which is an add-on code (and exempt from modifier -51).

ASSIGNMENT 12.2 – CODING PRACTICE

	ICD Codes	CPT Codes
1.	727.03	26055-F2
NOTE: To locate CPT code 26055, locate main term *Trigger finger repair* in the index.		
2.	518.89	31628
NOTE:		

NOTE:
- Assign code 518.89 for mucosal lesion of the bronchus because bronchi are branching passageways of the lungs. (Do not assign a code for hemoptysis, which is a symptom of the diagnosed mucosal lesion of the bronchus.
- The diagnostic bronchoscopy is included in the surgical bronchoscopy code.

	ICD Codes	CPT Codes
3.	V54.01	20680-LT

NOTE: To assign code V54.01, use the ICD-9-CM Index to Diseases and locate main term *Removal (of)*, subterm *device*, 2nd qualifier *fixation*, and 3rd qualifier *internal*.

4.	812.43	24575-LT

NOTE:
- To assign the ICD diagnosis code, locate main term *Fracture* and subterms *humerus, condyle* in the alphabetic index.
- The abbreviation for millimeters of mercury is mmHg.
- ORIF is the abbreviation for open reduction with internal fixation.

	ICD Codes	CPT Codes
5.	162.3	32480, 31622-51

NOTE:

- Do not assign a CPT code for insertion of a chest tube (code 32551) because the code description includes the phrase *separate procedure*. This means that the placement of chest tubes for drainage is considered an integral part of a thoracostomy with biopsy procedure.
- After the thoracostomy was performed, the patient underwent diagnostic bronchoscopy which is separately coded as 31622. Modifier -51 is added to this code to reflect that multiple procedures were performed during the same operative session.

6.	735.0, 726.91	28296-T5, 28288-51-T6

NOTE:

- Both ICD codes medically justify the procedure performed.
- According to the *CPT Assistant*, code 28296 is reported for an Austin, Chevron, or Mitchell bunionectomy.

7.	471.8	31032-RT
8.	212.1	31541
9.	784.7, E917.0	30905-LT, 30903-59-RT

NOTE:

- The patient underwent posterior packing and cautery, which is assigned CPT code 30905.
- The patient also underwent anterior packing after failed cautery on the right, which is assigned code 30903 to reflect a more complex treatment. Modifiers -59 (distinct procedure) and -RT are added to the code.

10.	518.82, 335.20	31600

NOTE:

- ALS is the abbreviation for amyotrophic lateral sclerosis, which is also known as Lou Gehrig's disease.
- Code 518.82 medically justifies the procedure performed. Code 335.20 is also reported because the condition contributed to the first-listed diagnosis.

REVIEW

Multiple Choice

1. c   2. c   3. b

Note:

The cast application is included in the definitive treatment code.

4. a   7. c   10. a
5. c   8. d   11. c
6. c   9. d   12. b

Note:

When a diagnostic laryngoscopy is performed during the same operative session as a surgical laryngoscopy, code only the surgical laryngoscopy. The diagnostic laryngoscopy is included in the surgical laryngoscopy code.

13. a   15. a   16. b
14. c

Note:

The fascia level is located below the subcutaneous level of skin.

17. d   18. a   19. c

Note:

The code description for 32500 indicates that the code is assigned if one wedge resection is done or if multiple wedge resections are done.

20. a

Chapter 13
CPT Surgery III

ASSIGNMENT 13.1 – CODING PRACTICE

	ICD Codes	CPT Codes
1.	454.9	37722-LT
2.	785.6	38510
3.	426.0	33210, 71090
4.	785.6	38570
5.	V46.11	36620

NOTE: Because no disease or condition was documented to justify respirator care, assign an ICD V code by locating main term *Status* in the alphabetic index.

6.	785.6	38720
7.	397.0	33464

NOTE: To assign the ICD diagnosis code, locate main term *Regurgitation* and subterm *tricuspid*. Note that the directional term see refers you to *Endocarditis, tricuspid.*

8.	572.3	38100
9.	996.04	33241, 33243-51, 33249-51

NOTE: To assign the ICD diagnosis code, locate main term *Complication*, subterm *device*, and qualifiers *cardiac* and *automatic implantable defibrillator.*

10.	289.59	38115

ASSIGNMENT 13.2 – CODING OPERATIVE REPORTS

	ICD Codes	CPT Codes
1.	426.0, 427.89, 412	33210, 71090

NOTE: This report documents the insertion of a temporary pacemaker electrode. It does not document or state that a permanent pacemaker with a pulse generator component was inserted.

2.	174.9	36558, 177001

NOTE: Tunneled catheters are placed through the skin in the middle of the chest. They are tunneled through the subcutaneous tissue and inserted into the superior vena cava vessel at the entrance of the right atrium of the heart. Tunneled catheters can be left in place for months or years with a low rate of infection. (Nontunneled catheters are inserted directly through the skin into the jugular or subclavian vein and are moved through the vein to the superior vena cava. Nontunneled catheters can be inserted at the bedside in a nonsurgical setting, and they are commonly used for short-term or emergency situations. Nontunneled catheters are also referred to as jugular or subclavian catheters.)

3.	V58.81	36589

NOTE: The patient was admitted for the removal of her Hickman catheter because symptoms associated with hyperemesis gravidarum had resolved. The ICD diagnosis code can be located by referring to main term *Removal* and subterms *catheter, vascular.* A Hickman catheter is a tunneled central venous (vascular) catheter, which means that it is inserted (or tunneled) under the skin and placed in a vein. (The purpose of tunneling the catheter under the skin is to help prevent infection.)

	ICD Codes	CPT Codes
4.	414.01	33535, 33518

NOTE:
- There is no documentation that the patient had previously undergone bypass surgery; therefore, ICD diagnosis code 414.01 is assigned.
- Code 33535 reflects the grafting of three arterial vessels.
- The saphenous vein was used for two grafts; therefore, CPT code 33518 is assigned.
- Cardioplegia and bypass are integral parts of a CABG, and they are not coded separately. (CABG is the abbreviation for coronary artery bypass graft.)

	ICD Codes	CPT Codes
5.	420.90	33010, 76930
6.	785.6	38525-LT
7.	289.59	38120

NOTE: Because a laparoscopic spleen removal procedure was documented, code 38120 is assigned (and not code 38100).

8.	683	38300
9.	202.83	38570

NOTE: The biopsied lymph nodes were located in the retroperitoneal area, which is the area behind the abdominal wall. Thus, a fifth digit 3 is assigned to the ICD diagnosis code.

10.	V59.3	38230

NOTE: To assign the ICD diagnosis code, locate main term *Donor* in the alphabetic index.

REVIEW

Multiple Choice

1. c

> **Note:**
>
> It is incorrect to assign modifier -63 to the CPT code. There is a note that directs the coder not to report modifier -63 with the code.

2. d	7. b	12. a
3. b	8. a	13. b
4. c	9. a	14. b
5. d	10. c	
6. d	11. c	

> **Note:**
>
> RBC is the abbreviation for red blood cell, and WBC is the abbreviation for white blood cell.

15. d	17. c	19. a
16. b	18. a	20. c

Chapter 14
CPT Surgery IV

ASSIGNMENT 14.1 – CODING PRACTICE

	ICD Codes	CPT Codes
1.	786.6	39000
2.	211.3	45385
3.	573.9	47000, 76942

NOTE: To assign the ICD diagnosis code, locate main term *Disease* and subterm *liver* in the alphabetic index. (Do not go to main term *Mass* and subterm *liver* because no code is found there. However, main term *Mass* and subterm *specified disease* directs the coder to the main term *Disease*.)

4.	599.70	52000
5.	553.21	49560

NOTE: This case documents that the patient has an incisional hernia.

6.	212.6	39400
7.	223.3	52204
8.	560.81, 197.7, V10.05	44005

NOTE: To locate ICD code 560.81, locate main term *Obstruction* and subterm *intestinal with adhesions.*

9.	212.6	39220
10.	565.0	46200
11.	553.3	39520
12.	599.70	52606
13.	098.0	53200

NOTE: To locate the ICD diagnosis code, locate main term *Urethritis* and subterm *gonococcal* in the alphabetic index.

14.	780.60	51100
15.	198.89, 199.1	39560

NOTE: This case documents cancer of the diaphragm as metastatic. To assign an ICD code to the unknown primary site, go to the Neoplasm Table and locate code 199.1 under the Secondary Malignancy column. (ICD code 199.1 is assigned as a secondary code to reflect that the primary neoplasm has a site that is not known in this case.)

ASSIGNMENT 14.2 – CODING OPERATIVE REPORTS

	ICD Codes	CPT Codes
1.	552.20, 553.1	49561, 49585-51

NOTE:
- For ICD coding purposes, the term *incarcerated* as documented in this report means "obstruction."
- The patient's age must be known to select the appropriate CPT code for an umbilical hernia repair.

2.	540.9	44950
3.	557.0, 537.89	49002

NOTE: This patient underwent a laparotomy one week prior to the laparotomy documented in this report.

285

ICD Codes	CPT Codes
4. 211.3	44140

NOTE: Another term for a hemicolectomy is a partial colectomy.

| 5. 550.10 | 49496-RT |

NOTE: The age of the patient must be known to assign the appropriate CPT code. Another factor important to assigning the correct CPT code is documentation of the incarcerated small bowel.

| 6. 236.7, 239.4 | 52235, 52332-51, 74420 |

NOTE:
- The physician identified the bladder tumor as a papilloma, which is assigned code 236.7 (papilloma). If a pathology report was not available, documentation from the operative report would be used to assign the ICD diagnosis code.
- A second bladder tumor was documented in the operative report, which is assigned code 239.4 (unspecified nature).
- Insertion of an indwelling stent is assigned an additional procedure code. If the stent was not indwelling or had not been left in place at the conclusion of the procedure, a separate code would not be assigned.
- According to *CPT Assistant,* code 74420 is reported once for the bilateral retrograde pyelograms and modifier -50 is not added to the code. According to Ingenix's Encoder Pro Expert software, directional modifiers (e.g., -LT and -RT) are also not added to the code.

| 7. 594.1, 591 | 52353, 52332-51 |

NOTE:
- The size of the bladder stone determines the correct CPT code.
- The insertion of an indwelling stent is coded as an additional procedure code. If the stent was not indwelling or was not left in place at the conclusion of the procedure, it would not be separately coded.

| 8. 592.1 | 52320-52 |

NOTE: Modifier -52 is added to the CPT code to identify a reduced service for a surgical procedure that was attempted but not completed.

| 9. 188.4 | 52224 |

NOTE:
- ICD code 188.4 is assigned for carcinoma of the bladder because documentation in the operative report indicates a posterior location.
- The site of the bladder tumor was not documented in the operative report, which means that the lowest code in range 52224–52240 is assigned. (The physician should be queried to provide information on the size of the tumor fulgurated on this patient.)

| 10. 592.1 | 52330, 74485 |

NOTE:
- The patient underwent manipulation of the ureteral stone in his bladder. Because the stone was not removed, CPT code 52330 is assigned.
- Ureteral fluoroscopy was performed to confirm the catheter's position during the operative procedure; ureteral fluoroscopy is included in CPT code 52330. Do not report a separate CPT code for ureteral fluoroscopy.
- Contrast material was injected into the catheter, and the entire left ureter and renal collecting system were outlined. Then dilatation of the ureter and collecting system was performed, which revealed presences of ureteral calculus. The fluoroscopically guided dilatation procedure is assigned CPT code 74485. (According to Ingenix's Encoder Pro Expert, directional modifiers -LT and -RT are not added to code 74485.)

| 11. 553.3 | 39502 |
| 12. 782.0, 719.40 | 39400 |

NOTE: The diagnosis "sarcoidosis" is unconfirmed at the time of the procedure, which means that ICD codes for the patient's reported symptoms are assigned.

13. 862.0	39501
14. 748.8	39200
15. 786.2	39010

NOTE:
- Because the diagnosis of lung carcinoma was not established at the time of surgery, an ICD code for the patient's symptom of cough is assigned.
- Chamberlain is an eponym for a mediastinotomy procedure, which involves incision in the third intercostal space or transthoracic space.

| 16. 239.0, 527.2 | 42415 |

REVIEW

Multiple Choice

1. b   3. b   4. b
2. d

Note:

ERCP is the abbreviation for endoscopic retrograde cholangiopancreatography.

5. d

Note:

EGD is the abbreviation for esophagogastroduodenoscopy.

6. c   7. a   8. a

Note:

- *A TURP includes a vasectomy, meatotomy, cystourethroscopy, urethral calibration, dilation, and/or internal urethrotomy. Codes for these procedures, when performed during the same operative session as a TURP, are not reported separately.*
- *TURP is the abbreviation for transurethral resection of the prostate.*

9. d   12. d   15. c
10. b   13. a   16. a
11. b   14. b

Note:

Cystoscopy is also known as cystourethroscopy.

17. b   19. d   20. d
18. a

Chapter 15
CPT Surgery V

ASSIGNMENT 15.1 – CODING PRACTICE

	ICD Codes	CPT Codes
1.	186.9	54520-LT
2.	246.2	60300-RT
3.	956.5	64834-RT, 69990

NOTE: To assign the ICD diagnosis code, locate main term *Injury*, subterm *nerve*, 2nd qualifier *foot*, and 3rd qualifier *specified site NEC* in the alphabetic index. (If main term *Laceration* and subterm *nerve* are referenced instead, the coder is directed to main term *Injury*.)

4.	650, V27.0	59400

NOTE:
- OB is the abbreviation for obstetrician.
- OA is the abbreviation for occipitoanterior.
- This is a delivery case, and ICD coding guidelines require the assignment of an outcome of delivery code to represent the status of the infant delivered. To assign this code, locate main term *Outcome* in the alphabetic index.
- This case documents that the physician provided antepartum, postpartum, and delivery care, which means that CPT code 59400 is assigned.

5.	245.2	60271

NOTE: Do not assign CPT code 60240 (Thyroidectomy, total or complete) because a cervical approach was used to perform the surgery, which is classified as code 60271.

6.	368.13	65430-LT
7.	233.5	54100

NOTE: To assign the ICD diagnosis code, locate main term *Bowen's*. The coder is directed to the Neoplasm Table and subterms *skin, penis, in situ.*

8.	623.8	57135
9.	356.9	64555
10.	346.90, 346.70	64405
11.	621.8	58520

NOTE: Do not mistakenly assign CPT code 59350, which classifies hysterorrhaphy of ruptured uterus for Maternal Care and Delivery. Code 58520 correctly classifies nonobstetrical hysterorrhaphy.

12.	921.2	67415, 77002-51

NOTE:
- To assign the ICD diagnosis code, locate main term *Hematoma*, subterm *orbit*, and 2nd qualifier *traumatic* in the alphabetic index.
- This case documents the use of a fluoroscope, which means that CPT code 77002 is assigned as an additional code.

13.	V55.8	69424-50

NOTE:
- To locate code V55.8, refer to main term *Attention* to and subterm *artificial opening (of)* in the ICD-9-CM Index to Diseases because the reason for the procedure is to remove previously placed ventilation tubes.
- This case documents removal of tubes from the right and left ear; therefore, modifier -50 is added to the CPT code.

14.	608.4	55100
15.	605, 607.1	54161
16.	252.00	60500

	ICD Codes	CPT Codes
17.	606.1	55300
18.	784.2	60210

NOTE: To assign the ICD diagnosis code, locate main term *Mass* and subterm *neck* in the ICD-9-CM Index to Diseases.

19.	227.5	60600
20.	380.4	69210

NOTE: The description of CPT code 69210 states one or both ears; therefore, modifier -50 is not added the CPT code.

21.	370.00	65450-LT

NOTE: A "corneal lesion" is a corneal ulcer and are commanly caused by trauma. Main term is ulcer subterm is cornea in ICD-9-CM index.

22.	641.01, V27.0	59514

NOTE:
- Apgar is named after anesthesiologist Virginia Apgar, and the acronym stands for activity, pulse, grimace, appearance, and respiration. It is an assessment of newborns typically at 1 minute and 5 minutes of birth. Each area (activity, pulse, etc) is assigned a score of 0, 1, or 2. The five areas are combined to achieve a total score. A total score of 7 to 10 is normal.
- This case documents a delivery, which means that an outcome of delivery ICD code (V27.0) is assigned.
- NICU is the abbreviation for neonatal intensive care unit.

23.	354.0	64721-LT
24.	173.2	69100

NOTE: To assign code 173.2, refer to the Neoplasm Table in the ICD-9-CM Index to Diseases and locate subterm *ear (external)*. Then locate code 173.2 in the Malignant, Primary column. (If main term *Carcinoma* is referenced, the coder is directed to the Neoplasm Table.)

25.	626.8	57180
26.	351.8	64732

NOTE: To assign code 351.8, locate main term *Neuritis* and subterm *facial* in the ICD-9-CM Index to Diseases. Notice that there is no subterm for *orbital*, *supraorbital*, or *frontal*. The supraorbital nerve is a branch of the frontal nerve, which passes through the supraorbital notch of the forehead. It controls sensory functions of the upper eyelid, eyebrow, forehead, scalp up to the occipital bone, and conjunctiva. It is classified as a facial nerve.

27.	365.22	66762
28.	634.91	59812

NOTE: In ICD, a miscarriage is a spontaneous abortion.

29.	216.1	67850-E1
30.	614.4	58823
31.	385.30	69540
32.	634.90	59425
33.	380.10	69020
34.	131.01	57105
35.	744.59	69300-LT

ASSIGNMENT 15.2 – CODING OPERATIVE REPORTS

	ICD Codes	CPT Codes
1.	185	52601

NOTE:
- TURP is an abbreviation for transurethral resection of the prostate.
- Cystoscopy is a diagnostic procedure that would not be coded or reported separately.

2.	600.00	55700, 76872
3.	V25.2	55250

NOTE: This patient was admitted for the sterilization procedure. To assign the ICD diagnosis code, locate main term *Admission*.

ICD Codes	CPT Codes
4. 603.9	55040

NOTE: According to Ingenix's Encoder Pro Expert software, directional modifiers (e.g., -LT and -RT) are not added to the CPT code.

5. 198.82	54520-50

NOTE: The patient has metastatic carcinoma from the prostate gland to the testicles. There is no documentation that the patient had previous prostatectomy or is undergoing chemotherapy or radiation treatment for the primary site. If this information was provided, ICD code 185 would be assigned to classify the primary prostate cancer (still under treatment or not removed). If documentation was present that the patient had previously undergone a prostatectomy and was no longer receiving treatment for prostate cancer, ICD code V10.46 could be assigned to reflect the patient's history of malignant neoplasm.

6. 618.6	57268
7. 218.9	58150, 44950-51-52

NOTE: This operative report documents that the patient's appendix was also removed. There is no documentation that the appendix was diseased; therefore, it is coded as an incidental appendectomy. Modifiers -51 (additional procedure) and -52 (reduced services) are added to the appendectomy code.

8. 626.9, V13.29	58120, 58661-50-51

NOTE: CPT code 58120 is reported for dilation and curettage of the endometrium of this patient. CPT code 58661 is reported for removal of the patient's fallopian tubes, which was done bilaterally. Modifiers -50 (bilateral procedure) and -51 (additional procedure) are added to the laparoscopic salpingectomy, bilateral, code.

9. 654.21, V27.0	59514

NOTE:
- An outcome of delivery code is assigned for the single liveborn infant.
- If this physician had provided routine antepartum and postpartum care, CPT code 59510 would have been assigned instead of 59514.
- Treatment of omentum adhesions is not separately coded unless lysis of adhesions takes significant time and effort and is reflected in the operative note as being extensive.

10. 642.41, V27.0	59514

NOTE: If this physician had provided routine antepartum and postpartum care, CPT code 59510 would have been assigned instead of 59514.

11. 650, V27.0	59409

NOTE:
- The bradycardia condition was not treated and is not assigned an ICD diagnosis code.
- If this physician had provided routine antepartum and postpartum care, CPT code 59400 would have been assigned instead of 59409.
- The episiotomy, including repair, and artificial rupture of membranes are included in code 59409. Do not assign separate CPT codes for these procedures.

12. 226	60220-RT

NOTE: This report documents a thyroid lobectomy procedure performed.

13. 351.8	64732
14. 355.6	64776-LT
15. 998.89	62100, 69990

NOTE:
- This report documents a complication of surgical care. To assign the ICD diagnosis code, locate main term *Complication* in the alphabetic index.
- Make sure you assign CPT code 69990 to indicate use of the operating microscope during surgery. The operating microscope code is an add-on code; therefore, modifier -51 (additional procedure) is not added to the code.

REVIEW

Multiple Choice

1. b   2. c   3. b

> **Note:**
>
> *The medical term for the condition ingrown eyelashes is trichiasis.*

4. c	8. d	12. d
5. a	9. a	13. c
6. b	10. d	
7. b	11. c	

Note:

The operating microscope code is an add-on code; therefore, modifier -51 (additional procedure) is not added to the code.

14. a	16. a	17. c
15. b		

Note:

The lesion was removed using cryosurgery; therefore, code 54056 is assigned. If the lesion had been excised, code 11421 could have been assigned.

18. c	19. b	20. c

Note:

This procedure was performed on an infant; however, the note states that modifier -63 is not assigned to codes 63704 and 63706.

Chapter 16
CPT Radiology

ASSIGNMENT 16.1 – CODING PRACTICE

	ICD Codes	CPT Codes
1.	789.01	76700
2.	724.2, E881.1, E849.3	72040, 72110

NOTE:
• No fracture was found on x-ray; therefore, assign an ICD code to the symptom only.

3.	786.50	71100-RT
4.	719.41, V54.89	73100-LT, 73030-LT
5.	786.05	71020
6.	526.9	70100
7.	794.8	78216
8.	722.10	72131
9.	719.42	73070-LT
10.	812.01	73030-LT

NOTE: When a fracture is not stated as open or closed, coding guidelines direct the coder to classify the fracture as closed.

11.	813.44	73110-LT
12.	786.50	71010
13.	719.45	72170
14.	787.20	74230
15.	789.00	74022

NOTE: Do not code the single view chest x-ray separately because it is included in CPT code 74022.

16.	784.2	70487

NOTE:
• A mass was found on radiological exam. To assign the ICD-9-CM diagnosis code for sinus mass, locate main term *Mass* and subterm *nose and sinus* in the alphabetic index.
• This case documents the use of a contrast agent, which means that CPT code 70487 is assigned.

17.	786.05, 786.50	71022
18.	620.2, 620.5	76856

NOTE: There is no documentation that this pelvic ultrasound was an obstetrical ultrasound. Therefore, refer to the nonobstetrical ultrasound code range (CPT codes 76830-76857). Documentation also supports the assignment of a complete code (instead of a limited or follow-up code).

19.	185	77327
20.	193	79403

ASSIGNMENT 16.2 – CODING RADIOLOGY REPORTS

	ICD Codes	CPT Codes
1.	722.4, 807.2	72040, 71020, 71120
2.	434.91, 784.3	70470
3.	786.50	71260
4.	794.4	74400

NOTE: To assign the CPT procedure code, locate main term *Urography* and subterm *intravenous* in the CPT index.

5.	747.81	77432, 70450
6.	789.06	74246
7.	786.50, 724.5, 473.0, 473.1, 789.2	71015, 70210, 74400
8.	786.50	78460
9.	789.1	76700
10.	438.11	70460

NOTE: Residual aphasia is classified in ICD-9-CM as a late effect. To assign the ICD-9-CM diagnosis code, locate main term *Late* in the alphabetic index.

11.	493.90	71030
12.	816.01	73120-LT

NOTE:
- To assign the ICD-9-CM diagnosis code, locate main term *Fracture* and subterm *phalanges* in the alphabetic index.
- According to Ingenix's Encoder Pro Expert, modifier -LT (or -RT) is added to code 73120. HCPCS level II modifier(s) specifying digits of the hand are not added to the code.

13.	782.0, 723.1	72240
14.	807.02, 733.00, 786.50, 719.45	72170, 73500-LT, 71010, 71100-LT
15.	240.9	70360
16.	794.4	74420
17.	553.3, 532.90, 562.00	74245
18.	346.90	70450
19.	241.1	78006
20.	733.00	73562-LT

REVIEW

Multiple Choice

1. c	6. b	11. d
2. c	7. b	12. b
3. b	8. d	13. d
4. d	9. b	14. c
5. a	10. c	

Note:

According to CPT, ribbons are considered temporary interstitial placement during clinical brachytherapy.

15. b   17. a   18. a
16. b

> **Note:**
>
> The abbreviation r/o means "rule out."

19. b

> **Note:**
>
> Because the physician provided an interpretation and report only, modifier -26 is added to the code.

20. c

Chapter 17
CPT Pathology and Laboratory

ASSIGNMENT 17.1 – CODING PRACTICE

	ICD Codes	CPT Codes
1.	783.21	80076, 85027

NOTE:
- ALT is the abbreviation for alanine aminotransferase (or transferase alanine amino as stated in the CPT coding manual), AST is the abbreviation for aspartate aminotransferase (or transferase aspartate amino as stated in the CPT coding manual), and CBC is the abbreviation for complete blood count.
- The albumin, bilirubin total and direct, phosphatase, protein, ALT, and AST tests constitute a panel code (CPT code 80076); however, this panel does not include a CBC. Therefore, code 80076 is also assigned.

2.	V70.8	86022

NOTE: To assign the diagnosis code, locate main term *Examination* and subterm *donor (potential)* in the ICD-9-CM Index to Diseases.

3.	780.79	88371
4.	659.53	88271

NOTE:
- Fluorescent in situ hybridization can be abbreviated as FISH.
- Gravida indicates the number of times this patient has been pregnant including the current pregnancy, and para indicates how many times the patient has delivered one or more fetuses. In this case, because the patient is gravida 1, para 0, she is still pregnant. Thus, fifth digit 3 is assigned to code 659.5x.
- Because the patient is age 46, she is considered an elderly primigravida.

5.	474.10	88304

NOTE:
- To assign the ICD-9-CM diagnosis code, the coder is directed by the alphabetic index to a combination code that reflects enlarged tonsils and adenoids.
- Tonsils and adenoids are located in level III of the surgical pathology codes in the Pathology and Laboratory section of CPT.

6.	782.1, 285.9	86039
7.	787.91	87045
8.	786.05, 780.79	88237
9.	599.70	88305

NOTE: Kidneys are located under level IV of the surgical pathology codes in the Pathology and Laboratory section of CPT.

10.	V70.5	80100
11.	V72.83	80061, 82947

NOTE:
- CPT classifies total cholesterol, HDL, and triglycerides as a lipid panel.
- HDL is the abbreviation for high density lipoproteins.

12.	788.41	87086
13.	225.0	88037
14.	197.7	88307

NOTE:
- To assign the ICD-9-CM diagnosis code, go to the Neoplasm Table in the alphabetic index and locate the secondary column (for metastatic) under the Malignant columns.
- The liver is located under level V of the surgical pathology codes in the Pathology and Laboratory section of CPT.

	ICD Codes	CPT Codes
15.	V73.3	86762

NOTE: To assign the ICD-9-CM diagnosis code, locate main term *Screening* and subterm *rubella* in the alphabetic index.

	ICD Codes	CPT Codes
16.	V81.5	82565

NOTE:
- To assign the ICD-9-CM diagnosis code, locate main term *Screening* and subterm *renal disease* in the alphabetic index.
- The renal insufficiency diagnosis was not confirmed as a disease, and it is incorrect to assign ICD-9-CM diagnosis code 593.9.

	ICD Codes	CPT Codes
17.	V72.31	88142
18.	783.43	86277
19.	606.9	89321
20.	704.00	87101

ASSIGNMENT 17.2 – CODING PATHOLOGY AND LABORATORY REPORTS

	ICD Codes	CPT Codes
1.	786.50	82550, 83625

NOTE: Cardiac isoenzymes test CPK and LDH levels in blood serum and help determine the location of tissue damage, such as heart tissue. CPK is the abbreviation for creatine phosphokinase, and LDH is the abbreviation for lactate (or lactic) dehydrogenase.

	ICD Codes	CPT Codes
2.	780.79	85027

NOTE: Because this CBC laboratory test did not include a differential WBC count, CPT code 85027 is assigned (instead of 85025).

	ICD Codes	CPT Codes
3.	V08	87075
4.	788.1	81005
5.	518.82	82805
6.	782.1	86592
7.	532.50	87070
8.	788.1, 599.70	87086
9.	496	82803
10.	595.9	88305

NOTE: To assign the CPT procedure code, locate main term *Urinary bladder* and subterm *biopsy* in the alphabetic index.

	ICD Codes	CPT Codes
11.	685.0	88304
12.	V25.2	88302

NOTE: CPT code 88302 reflects the fallopian tube submitted as a part of sterilization procedure.

	ICD Codes	CPT Codes
13.	366.9	88300
14.	780.8	80053, 82465, 84550

NOTE: The CPT panel code does not include the uric acid and cholesterol laboratory tests, which are assigned separate codes.

	ICD Codes	CPT Codes
15.	719.50	85025

NOTE: Assign CPT code 85025 to a complete blood count (CBC) with differential (not code 85027).

	ICD Codes	CPT Codes
16.	V72.83	81007
17.	226	88307
18.	634.91	88305

NOTE: Fifth digit 1 identifies the incomplete condition in ICD-9-CM code 634.91.

	ICD Codes	CPT Codes
19.	709.2, V54.01	88304, 88300

NOTE:
- To assign diagnosis code 709.2, locate main term *Scar* in the ICD-9-CM Index to Diseases.
- To assign diagnosis code V54.01, locate main term *Removal*, subterm *device*, 2nd qualifier *fixation*, and 3rd qualifier *internal*. (The patient underwent surgery to remove the metal rod from his hip.)
- CPT code 88304 is assigned for gross and microscopic examination of scar from left lower leg and debridement tissue. CPT code 88300 is assigned for gross examination of the metal rod that was removed.

| 20. | 594.1 | 88300 |

REVIEW

Multiple Choice

1. a

> **Note:**
>
> *Hep is the abbreviation for hepatitis.*

2. c	5. c	8. c
3. b	6. b	9. d
4. a	7. c	

> **Note:**
>
> *CPT code 80048 is assigned for a basic metabolic blood panel only when all laboratory tests associated with the panel are performed. In this case, because just three of the tests were performed, a separate CPT code is assigned for each.*

10. b	12. c	14. c
11. c	13. d	15. d

> **Note:**
>
> *Chickenpox is also known as varicella zoster.*

16. b
17. b

> **Note:**
>
> *Sed is the abbreviation for sedimentation.*

18. a
19. a
20. d

Chapter 18
CPT Medicine

ASSIGNMENT 18.1 – CODING PRACTICE

	ICD Codes	CPT Codes
1.	492.8	94621
2.	368.8, 250.00	92235
3.	V56.0, 787.02, 780.4	90937
4.	174.9	96413, 96415

NOTE: CPT code 96415 is an add-on code that reflects the additional hours of chemotherapy treatment via infusion. Modifier -51 is not added to add-on codes.

	ICD Codes	CPT Codes
5.	311	90847
6.	388.30	92625
7.	427.9	92960
8.	367.4	92342
9.	892.0	90471, 90703

NOTE:
- For ICD-9-CM coding purposes, a retained foreign object or foreign body is classified as a complicated open wound. However, in this case, the patient removed the object (needle) and brought it with him to the clinic.
- CPT code 90471 is assigned for the administration of the injection via intramuscular (IM) route, and code 90703 is assigned for the vaccine (that is located in the syringe).
- Because this patient is over age 7, code 90702 is not assigned.
- Because there is no documentation that this vaccine was preservative-free, code 90714 is not assigned.

	ICD Codes	CPT Codes
10.	V71.89	91105

NOTE: This child was lavaged due to suspected ingestion of a poison. However, documentation does not confirm that this case is a poisoning. Therefore, assign an ICD-9-CM diagnosis code for observation of specified suspected condition.

ASSIGNMENT 18.2 – CODING MEDICINE REPORTS

	ICD Codes	CPT Codes
1.	V81.2	93880
2.	780.39	95816
3.	784.3	92506
4.	786.59, 401.9, 414.00, 780.79, 780.4	93015

NOTE:
- METs is the abbreviation for metabolic equivalents.
- This patient has a documented history of chest discomfort and medical history of hypertension. During the exam, the patient experienced weakness and dizziness; therefore, codes for those symptoms are also assigned.

	ICD Codes	CPT Codes
5.	786.05	94660

NOTE: CPAP is the abbreviation for continuous positive airway pressure.

	ICD Codes	CPT Codes
6.	724.5, 782.0, 724.8	97001

NOTE:
- RLE is the abbreviation for right lower extremity, and RLQ is the abbreviation for right lower quadrant.
- For ICD-9-CM coding, because the patient complains of back pain and muscle spasms, codes are assigned for each. During the evaluation, the patient reported numbness, which is also coded.

	ICD Codes	CPT Codes
7.	244.9, 704.00	96902
8.	250.01	96522
9.	746.3	93315

NOTE:
- TEE is the abbreviation for transesophageal echocardiography, and NICU is the abbreviation for neonatal intensive care unit.
- This test was performed on a 5-day-old infant, which means that the ICD-9-CM diagnosis code for congenital aortic stenosis code is assigned (not the acquired code number, 424.1).
- E codes are not usually assigned for outpatient encounters.

	ICD Codes	CPT Codes
10.	787.01	91132

REVIEW

Multiple Choice

1. c

Note:

IM is the abbreviation for intramuscular.

2. b   3. b   4. b   5. b

Note:

Although five manipulations were performed, just three regions were manipulated.

6. c   7. c

Note:

ESRD is the abbreviation for end-stage renal disease.

8. d

9. b

Note:

SAECG is the abbreviation for signal-averaged electrocardiography. Modifier –26 is added to CPT code 93278 to report the physician interpretation and reporting.

10. b
11. c

12. a
13. d

14. a
15. b

> **Note:**
>
> *HepA is the abbreviation for hepatitis A, and HepB is the abbreviation for hepatitis B.*

16. d
17. a

18. d
19. b

20. b

Chapter 19
Insurance and Reimbursement

ASSIGNMENT 19.1 – CHARGEMASTER REVIEW PROCESS

1. No, the street address is missing.
2. No, the chargemaster is dated April 5, YYYY.
3. Yes, the service descriptions listed in Column 2 describe services provided by the radiology department.
4. No.
   - Code 71012 should be changed to 71020.
   - Code 71034 is for four views.
   - Code 74214 should be changed to 74241.
   - Code 74274 is not a valid code.
   - Code 74250 does not have "separate procedure" in its CPT description.
5. Yes.

ASSIGNMENT 19.2 – INTERPRETING A REMITTANCE ADVICE

1. The check number is 9568547, and the amount is $905.
2. 0405YY
3. $20
4. When the student looks up the CPT code for Joseph Lynch's visit, he or she will see that it is a code for preventive services. The student could determine that the payer requires no coinsurance payment for preventive services.
5. FISC1234567-01
6. Each patient had a place of service (POS) code of 11.
7. 99212
8. $905
9. $60
10. $750

ASSIGNMENT 19.3 – INTERPRETING A MEDICARE FEE-FOR-SERVICE PAYMENT ERROR REPORT

1. Yes, FY 2004 is down by 1.3 percent in the Insufficient Documentation category. The area of nonresponse increased from FY 2003 at 18.5 percent to FY 2004 at 29.7 percent, which is an increase of 11.2 percent.
2. c
3. Yes, this category has seen improvement. In FY 2002, the percentage was 14.3; and in FY 2004, the percentage was 7.7, which is a decrease of 6.6 percent.

4. When comparing FY 2004 to FY 2003, the medically unnecessary type of error improved, decreasing by 4.5 percent (from 21.7 percent to 17.2 percent).

5. There is a decrease of 4.4 percent (12.1% to 7.7%).

ASSIGNMENT 19.4 – AMBULATORY PAYMENT CLASSIFICATIONS

1. a.

First-Listed diagnosis code:	553.1
Additional diagnosis code:	
Additional diagnosis code:	
Procedure code:	49585

b.
   i. 00154
   ii. $1690.75

2. a.

First-Listed diagnosis code:	599.70
Additional diagnosis code:	
Additional diagnosis code:	
Procedure code:	52000

b.
   i. 00160
   ii. $407.54

3. a.

First-Listed diagnosis code:	780.79
Additional diagnosis code:	794.5
Additional diagnosis code:	
Procedure code:	10021

b.
   i. 00002
   ii. $83.60

4. a.

First-Listed diagnosis code:	366.9
Additional diagnosis code:	
Additional diagnosis code:	
Procedure code:	66984-LT

b.
   i. 00246
   ii. $1405.02
   ii. $880.88

5. a.

First-Listed diagnosis code:	574.00
Additional diagnosis code:	574.10
Additional diagnosis code:	
Procedure code:	47563

b.
    i. 00131 and 00263. The APC of 00263 is for the intraoperative choliagogram.
    ii. $2686.08
    ii. $1733.39

ASSIGNMENT 19.5 – INTERPRETING DIAGNOSIS-RELATED GROUPS DECISION TREES

Medical Partitioning DRG Decision Tree (Figure 19-4 in the workbook)

1. DRG 14
2. DRG 19
3. DRG 18
4. DRG 11
5. DRG 17

Surgical Partitioning DRG Decision Tree (Figure 19-5 in the Workbook)

6. DRG 6
7. DRG 531
8. DRG 3
9. DRG 533
10. DRG 529

ASSIGNMENT 19.6 – ASSIGNING DIAGNOSIS-RELATED GROUPS

> **Note:**
>
> *Estimated Medicare reimbursement amounts included in each answer are based on the Medicare DRG calculator results at the IRP.com Web site. You may notice different reimbursement amounts if other DRG groupers (e.g., 3M or QuadraMed) are used and/or as the IRP.com Web site is updated to reflect revised case mix weights and other data.*

1a.

Principal diagnosis code:	428.0
Comorbidity code:	482.0
Comorbidity code:	404.91
Comorbidity code:	250.00
Comorbidity code:	272.4

Comorbidities of type 2 diabetes mellitus and hyperlipidemia were treated during this inpatient admission.

1b.
- 05
- 127 HEART FAILURE & SHOCK
- Estimated Medicare Reimbursement = $4,975.90

1c.
- 04
- 079 RESPIRATORY INFECTIONS & INFLAMMATIONS AGE >17 W CC

- Estimated Medicare Reimbursement = $7,810.41
- Either condition could be sequenced as the principal diagnosis based on the information presented in the case and ICD-9-CM coding guidelines.
- Yes. Changing the principal diagnosis from "congestive heart failure" to "pneumonia due to Klebsiella pneumoniae" increases the estimated DRG reimbursement amount.

2a.

Principal diagnosis code:	480.9
Comorbidity code:	438.82
Comorbidity code:	250.00
Comorbidity code:	401.9
Principal procedure code:	43.11

The patient's comorbidities of type 2 diabetes mellitus and hypertension were treated as an inpatient.

2b.

- 04
- 090 SIMPLE PNEUMONIA & PLEURISY AGE >17 W/O CC
- Estimated Medicare Reimbursement = $3,100.86

2c.

- 01
- 012 DEGENERATIVE NERVOUS SYSTEM DISORDERS
- Estimated Medicare Reimbursement = $4,589.99
- The late effect of cerebrovascular accident (CVA) with dysphagia should not be sequenced as the principal diagnosis because it was not treated during the inpatient admissions (e.g., speech therapy); viral pneumonia is the principal diagnosis.
- No. Changing the principal diagnosis to late effect of cerebrovascular accident (CVA) with dysphagia maximizes the DRG reimbursement rate, which is fraud. It is also an example of DRG creep.

3a.

Principal diagnosis code:	784.7
Comorbidity code:	285.1
Comorbidity code:	250.00
Comorbidity code:	401.9
Comorbidity code:	272.4
Principal procedure code:	21.03
Additional procedure code:	99.04

This patient's comorbidities of type 2 diabetes mellitus and hypertension were treated during this admission. All transfusions are coded on inpatient hospital stays due to training required to perform this procedure. Under UHDDS guidelines, all significant procedures that are surgical in nature carry an anesthetic risk; or if the procedures require specialized training to perform, they should be reported.

3b.

- 03
- 066EPISTAXIS
- Estimated Medicare Reimbursement = $2,944.61

3c.

- 16
- 395 RED BLOOD CELL DISORDERS AGE >17

- Estimated Medicare Reimbursement = $4,219.72
- The sequencing of diagnoses in 3c results in a higher estimated Medicare reimbursement.
- No. Changing the principal diagnosis to "acute posthemorrhagic anemia" maximizes the DRG reimbursement rate, which is fraud. It is also an example of DRG creep.

4a.

Principal diagnosis code:	996.73
Complication code:	403.91
Comorbidity code:	997.1
Comorbidity code:	E878.8
Principal procedure code:	39.50
Additional procedure code:	88.60

The sinus tachycardia developed postoperatively and is coded.

4b.

- 05
- 554 OTHER VASCULAR PROCEDURES W CC WITHOUT MAJOR CV DIAGNOSIS
- Estimated Medicare Reimbursement = $9,966.72

4c.

- 11
- 315 OTHER KIDNEY & URINARY TRACT PROCEDURES
- Estimated Medicare Reimbursement = $10,015.78
- The sequencing of diagnoses in 3c results in a higher estimated Medicare reimbursement.
- No. Changing the principal diagnosis to "hypertensive renal disease" maximizes the DRG reimbursement rate, which is fraud. It is also an example of DRG creep.

5a.

Principal diagnosis code:	424.1
Comorbidity code:	V45.81
Comorbidity code:	274.9
Comorbidity code:	V10.05
Principal procedure code:	35.22
Additional procedure code:	37.23

Assigning V codes for this case is valid. The patient's history of bypass surgery was a clinical reason for the cardiac catheterization procedure that was performed during this admission. The history of colon neoplasm code is reported for statistical purposes.

5b.

- 05
- 104 CARDIAC VALVE & OTHER MAJOR CARDIOTHORACIC PROC W CARDIAC CATH
- Estimated Medicare Reimbursement = $39,780.59

5c.

- 05
- 105 CARDIAC VALVE & OTHER MAJOR CARDIOTHORACIC PROC W/O CARDIAC CATH
- Estimated Medicare Reimbursement = $29,107.95
- The sequencing of diagnoses in 3c results in a higher estimated Medicare reimbursement.
- If the cardiac catheterization code is not reported, a loss of $10,672.64 results.

ASSIGNMENT 19.7 – RESOURCE UTILIZATION GROUPS

1. b

> **Note:**
>
> *Divide each RUG-53 category nonlabor rate into the total rate to calculate the approximately 24 percent. For example, RUX = 136/564.83 × 100 = 24%.*

2. c

> **Note:**
>
> *Divide each RUG-53 category labor rate into the total rate to calculate the approximately 76 percent. For example, RUX = 428.83/564.83 × 100 = 76%.*

3. c

> **Note:**
>
> *The total rate for RUC is $479.53, and the total rate for RUX is $564.83. The percentage increase from RUC to RUX is calculated by subtracting $479.53 from $564.83, dividing that calculated figure into $564.83, and multiplying by 100 to calculate the percentage. Thus,*
>
> - *479.53 − 564.83 = 85.30*
> - *85.30/564.83 = 0.1510*
> - *0.1510 × 100 = 15%*

4. Upon entry of all data, the student's spreadsheet should look similar to the following:

RUG-53 Category	Total Rate	Labor Portion	Nonlabor Portion
Rehabilitation Ultra High plus Extensive Services High (RUX)	564.83	428.83	136
Rehabilitation Ultra High plus Extensive Services Low (RUL)	496.04	376.6	119.44
Rehabilitation Very High plus Extensive Services High (RVX)	428.24	325.13	103.11
Rehabilitation Very High plus Extensive Services Low (RVL)	399.34	303.19	96.15
Rehabilitation High plus Extensive Services High (RHX)	363.02	275.61	87.41
Rehabilitation High plus Extensive Services Low (RHL)	356.14	270.39	85.75
Rehabilitation Medium (RMC)	308.25	234.03	74.22
Rehabilitation Medium (RMB)	299.99	227.76	72.23
Rehabilitation Medium (RMA)	293.11	222.53	70.58
Rehabilitation Low (RLB)	271.64	206.23	65.41
Rehabilitation Low (RLA)	231.74	175.94	55.8

5. Upon completion of the chart wizard, the student's pie chart should look similar to the following:

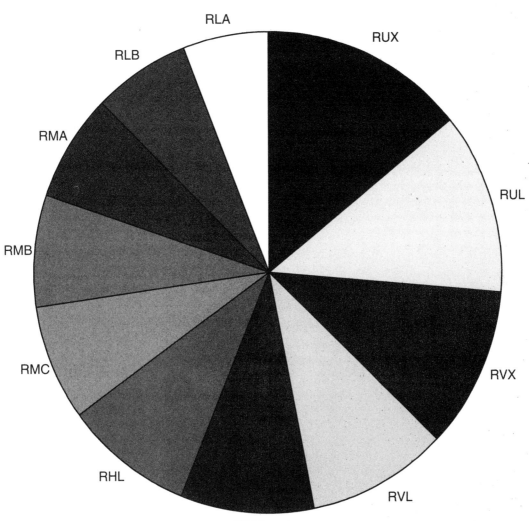

Total Rate

REVIEW

Multiple Choice

1. a	8. b	15. d
2. d	9. a	16. b
3. b	10. d	17. a
4. a	11. d	18. c
5. a	12. c	19. c
6. d	13. c	20. c
7. a	14. b	

Answer Keys to Workbook Coding Cases

CODING ANSWER KEYS

- Ambulatory Surgery Unit Coding Cases Answer Key (for Workbook Appendix A)
- Emergency Department Coding Cases Answer Key (for Workbook Appendix B)
- Physician Office Coding Cases Answer Key (for Workbook Appendix C)
- Inpatient Coding Cases Answer Key (for Workbook Appendix D)

Note:

Coding answers are from 2009 ICD-9-CM, CPT, and HCPCS level II.

Workbook Appendix A: Ambulatory Surgery Unit Coding Cases

ASUCASES ANSWER KEY

ASUCase001	Admission Diagnosis	First-Listed Diagnosis	Secondary Diagnosis	Secondary Diagnosis	Secondary Diagnosis
	354.0	354.0	727.05		
	First-Listed Procedure	Secondary Procedure	Secondary Procedure	Secondary Procedure	Secondary Procedure
	64721-RT	26145-51-F8	26145-F9	25115-51	

The reference to "4½ loupe magnification" is not microscopic surgery, which means that CPT code 64727 is not assigned in addition to code 64721-RT.

Add modifier -51 to the first reporting of secondary procedure code 26145, but not to subsequent reporting (due to the word "each" in the code description). A third-party payer knows to pay 26145 at a certain rate; and if the code (26145) is reported multiple times, the payer discounts subsequent reportings. Don't forget to add HCPCS alphanumeric modifiers (e.g., RT and F8) where appropriate. Report 26145-51-F8 for the right ring finger surgery and 26145-F9 for the right little finger surgery. (Reference to the ring and little fingers can be found in the operative report.)

Code 25115 is assigned to report tenosynovectomy of wrist, which is documented in the narrative of the operative report. Add modifier -51 to this code.

NOTE: Code 88305 would be assigned by the pathologist who examines tissue removed during surgery. Code 01810 would be assigned by the anesthesiologist.

ASUCase002	Admission Diagnosis	First-Listed Diagnosis	Secondary Diagnosis	Secondary Diagnosis	Secondary Diagnosis	Secondary Procedure
	622.11	622.11	623.8			
	First-Listed Procedure	Secondary Procedure	Secondary Procedure	Secondary Procedure	Secondary Procedure	Secondary Procedure
	57513	57010-51	80048	85027	85610	

CPT coding rules require reporting of chemistry panel code 80048 (Basic Metabolic, which covers calcium, CO2, chloride, creatinine, glucose, potassium, sodium, and BUN). CPT code 85027 is reported for a complete blood count (CBC), which includes WBC, RBC, Hgb, Hct, and platelets. Code 85610 is reported for the prothrombin time (PT).

ASUCase003	Admission Diagnosis	First-Listed Diagnosis	Secondary Diagnosis	Secondary Diagnosis	Secondary Diagnosis	Secondary Procedure
	724.4	724.4	729.1			
	First-Listed Procedure	Secondary Procedure	Secondary Procedure	Secondary Procedure	Secondary Procedure	Secondary Procedure
	64483					

To locate code 724.4, go to main term Radiculopathy in the ICD-9-CM Index to Diseases and follow the instruction to "see also Radiculitis." Then go to main term Radiculitis and subterm lumbosacral to locate code 724.4.

315

ASUCase004	Admission Diagnosis	First-Listed Diagnosis	Secondary Diagnosis			
	625.9	628.9	625.9			
	First-Listed Procedure	Secondary Procedure	Secondary Procedure	Secondary Procedure	Secondary Procedure	Secondary Procedure
	49320	80048	85027	85610		

Do not assign code 58350-51 for hydrotubation of uterus. Code 58350 is reported for chromotubation of oviduct (fallopian tube). Hydrotubation of the uterus is included as part of the diagnostic laparoscopy and not separately coded.

ASUCase005	Admission Diagnosis	First-Listed Diagnosis	Secondary Diagnosis	Secondary Diagnosis	Secondary Diagnosis	Secondary Procedure
	V25.2	V25.2	V58.69			
	First-Listed Procedure	Secondary Procedure	Secondary Procedure	Secondary Procedure	Secondary Procedure	Secondary Procedure
	58671	80048	85027	85610		

Code V58.69 is assigned for the documented long-term use of lithium.

ASUCase006	Admission Diagnosis	First-Listed Diagnosis	Secondary Diagnosis	Secondary Diagnosis	Secondary Diagnosis	Secondary Procedure
	654.53	654.53				
	First-Listed Procedure	Secondary Procedure	Secondary Procedure	Secondary Procedure	Secondary Procedure	Secondary Procedure
	59320	80048	85027	85610		

ICD code 654.53 is reported because this is an antepartum condition for a patient who is at 13 weeks' gestation. She previously had a 23-week loss of twins secondary to cervical incompetence; but that is in her past history, so code 654.54 (postpartum complication) is not reported.

ASUCase007	Admission Diagnosis	First-Listed Diagnosis				
	078.11	078.11				
	First-Listed Procedure	Secondary Procedure	Secondary Procedure	Secondary Procedure	Secondary Procedure	Secondary Procedure
	56620	80048	85027	85610		

CPT code 56620 (Vulvectomy, simple; partial) is reported for "vulvar excisional biopsy." Do not report a code from the CPT Integumentary section for that surgery.

ASUCase008	Admission Diagnosis	First-Listed Diagnosis	Secondary Diagnosis	Secondary Diagnosis	Secondary Diagnosis	Secondary Procedure
	620.2	620.2				
	First-Listed Procedure	Secondary Procedure	Secondary Procedure	Secondary Procedure	Secondary Procedure	Secondary Procedure
	58662	80048	85027	85610		

ASUCase009	Admission Diagnosis	First-Listed Diagnosis	Secondary Diagnosis	Secondary Diagnosis	Secondary Diagnosis	Secondary Procedure
	V54.01	V54.01				
	First-Listed Procedure	Secondary Procedure	Secondary Procedure	Secondary Procedure	Secondary Procedure	Secondary Procedure
	20680-RT	80048	85027	85610		

CPT code 88307 would be reported by the pathologist for gross and microscopic examination of specimen(s) removed during surgery.

ASUCase010	Admission Diagnosis	First-Listed Diagnosis	Secondary Diagnosis	Secondary Diagnosis	Secondary Diagnosis	Secondary Procedure
	727.03	727.03				
	First-Listed Procedure	Secondary Procedure	Secondary Procedure	Secondary Procedure	Secondary Procedure	Secondary Procedure
	26055-F2	80048	85027	85610		

Don't forget to add HCPCS modifier -F2 to indicate "middle finger."

Do not mistakenly assign code 26440-F2, which is reported for tenolysis of a trigger finger. This patient underwent incision of the tendon sheath to release the trigger finger. Per documentation in the operative report, the more invasive tenolysis procedure was not required.

Workbook Appendix B: Emergency Department Coding Cases

EDCASES ANSWER KEY

EDCase001	First-Listed Diagnosis	Secondary Diagnosis	Secondary Diagnosis	Secondary Diagnosis	Secondary Diagnosis	Secondary Diagnosis
	891.0	E920.8	E849.0			
	First-Listed Procedure	Secondary Procedure	Secondary Procedure	Secondary Procedure	Secondary Procedure	Secondary Procedure
	99281	90703	90471			
EDCase002	First-Listed Diagnosis	Secondary Diagnosis	Secondary Diagnosis	Secondary Diagnosis	Secondary Diagnosis	Secondary Diagnosis
	883.0	E920.8	E849.0			
	First-Listed Procedure	Secondary Procedure	Secondary Procedure	Secondary Procedure	Secondary Procedure	Secondary Procedure
	99281-25	12002-F6	90703	90471		

Do not assign ICD code V22.0 because the ED physician is not supervising the patient's pregnancy.
   Modifier -54 (Surgical Care Only) would be added to code 12002 if the ED physician provided surgical care only.

EDCase003	First-Listed Diagnosis	Secondary Diagnosis	Secondary Diagnosis	Secondary Diagnosis	Secondary Diagnosis	Secondary Diagnosis
	881.22	881.02	882.0	883.0	E920.8	E849.0
	First-Listed Procedure	Secondary Procedure	Secondary Procedure	Secondary Procedure	Secondary Procedure	Secondary Procedure
	99281-25	25260-RT	12001-59	90703	90471	

Coding guidelines indicate that tendon repair should be reported with a code associated with the appropriate system. Thus, code 25260-RT is reported for the tendon repair.
   Code 12001 is also reported for the simple repair of the additional wound that required suturing. Modifier -RT is not added to code 12001. (Do *not* report CPT code 12032, which is reported for wounds affecting the deeper layers of the subcutaneous tissue and nonmuscle fascia.)

EDCase004	First-Listed Diagnosis	Secondary Diagnosis	Secondary Diagnosis	Secondary Diagnosis	Secondary Diagnosis	Secondary Diagnosis
	870.8	368.8	E914	E917.9	E849.0	
	First-Listed Procedure	Secondary Procedure	Secondary Procedure	Secondary Procedure	Secondary Procedure	Secondary Procedure
	99282	90703	90471			
EDCase005	First-Listed Diagnosis	Secondary Diagnosis	Secondary Diagnosis	Secondary Diagnosis	Secondary Diagnosis	Secondary Diagnosis
	810.02	922.1	807.03	E820.0	E849.4	
	First-Listed Procedure	Secondary Procedure	Secondary Procedure	Secondary Procedure	Secondary Procedure	Secondary Procedure
	99282	71100	73000-RT	73030-RT	A4565	

Although the chest x-ray report documents "thickening of the pleura in this region suggesting associated hemorrhage," do not assign codes to these conditions because the emergency department (ED) physician did not document them on the face sheet. In the real world, a coder would generate a physician query to ask the ED physician if diagnoses should be added to the face sheet based on documentation in the x-ray report.

According to Ingenix's Encoder Pro Expert software, directional modifier -RT is not added to CPT code 71100, but it is added to codes 73000 and 73030. (After entering a CPT code in Encoder Pro Expert, click the M button on the toolbar to determine which modifiers can be added to the code.)

EDCase006	First-Listed Diagnosis	Secondary Diagnosis	Secondary Diagnosis	Secondary Diagnosis	Secondary Diagnosis	Secondary Diagnosis
	891.0	E880.9	E849.0			
	First-Listed Procedure	Secondary Procedure	Secondary Procedure	Secondary Procedure	Secondary Procedure 73562-RT	Secondary Procedure
	99281-25	12002	90471	90703		

Do not assign a CPT E/M code for this case because the ED physician did not document E/M services.

According to Ingenix's Encoder Pro Expert software, directional modifier -RT is not added to CPT code 12031.

Modifier -54 (Surgical Care Only) would be added to code 12031 if the ED physician provided surgical care only.

EDCase007	First-Listed Diagnosis	Secondary Diagnosis	Secondary Diagnosis	Secondary Diagnosis	Secondary Diagnosis	Secondary Diagnosis
	873.44	E885.9	E849.0			
	First-Listed Procedure	Secondary Procedure	Secondary Procedure	Secondary Procedure	Secondary Procedure	Secondary Procedure
	99281-25	12011				

EDCase008	First-Listed Diagnosis	Secondary Diagnosis	Secondary Diagnosis	Secondary Diagnosis	Secondary Diagnosis	Secondary Diagnosis
	873.0	924.4	923.8	E819.1		
	First-Listed Procedure	Secondary Procedure	Secondary Procedure	Secondary Procedure	Secondary Procedure	Secondary Procedure
	99282-25	12002	70260	90703	90471	

There is no CPT or HCPCS level II code for the oral administration of Tylenol. That service is included in the CPT E/M code (99283).

EDCase009	First-Listed Diagnosis	Secondary Diagnosis	Secondary Diagnosis	Secondary Diagnosis	Secondary Diagnosis	Secondary Diagnosis
	883.0	881.00	E920.8	E917.3	E849.0	
	First-Listed Procedure	Secondary Procedure	Secondary Procedure	Secondary Procedure	Secondary Procedure	Secondary Procedure
	12002					

When coding lacerations (12002), add like areas together that are treated using the same method and assign one CPT code. Do not assign separate codes for multiple lacerations of the same site.

Do not assign a CPT E/M service code for this case because the ED physician did not document provision of services.

The nurse's notes state that the patient's last tetanus shot was 6–7 years ago; there is no documentation that tetanus toxoid was administered during this encounter.

EDCase010	First-Listed Diagnosis	Secondary Diagnosis	Secondary Diagnosis	Secondary Diagnosis	Secondary Diagnosis	Secondary Diagnosis
	V58.43					
	First-Listed Procedure	Secondary Procedure	Secondary Procedure	Secondary Procedure	Secondary Procedure	Secondary Procedure
	99281					

This case is a recheck of a previously treated injury, which means that a V code is assigned.

Workbook Appendix C: Physician Office Coding Cases

POCASES ANSWER KEY

POCase001	First-Listed Diagnosis	Secondary Diagnosis	Secondary Diagnosis	Secondary Diagnosis	Secondary Diagnosis	Secondary Diagnosis
	296.40					
	First-Listed Procedure	Secondary Procedure	Secondary Procedure	Secondary Procedure	Secondary Procedure	Secondary Procedure
	99212	90862				

Report 296.40 because documentation indicates that this patient suffers from the manic type of bipolar disorder. The description in ICD for 296.4x indicates "most recent episode," and documentation in the patient's record is of manic type.

This provider is a psychiatrist, which is a medical doctor who reports appropriate level E/M codes for office visits. (If psychotherapy had been provided during the encounter in addition to or instead of an E/M service, the physician would also report an appropriate medicine code, such as code 90805.)

The statement in the notes "Patient seen today for regular appointment" indicates that this is an established patient. The levels of history and exam are problem focused, and medical decision making is straightforward.

POCase002	First-Listed Diagnosis	Secondary Diagnosis	Secondary Diagnosis	Secondary Diagnosis	Secondary Diagnosis	Secondary Diagnosis
	300.4	781.2				
	First-Listed Procedure	Secondary Procedure	Secondary Procedure	Secondary Procedure	Secondary Procedure	Secondary Procedure
	99212	90682				

This provider is a psychiatrist, which is a medical doctor who reports appropriate level E/M codes for office visits. (If psychotherapy had been provided during the encounter in addition to or instead of an E/M service, the physician would also report an appropriate medicine code, such as code 90805.)

The statement in the notes "Patient seen for regular appointment today" indicates that this is an established patient. The levels of history and exam are problem focused, and medical decision making is straightforward.

POCase003	First-Listed Diagnosis	Secondary Diagnosis	Secondary Diagnosis	Secondary Diagnosis	Secondary Diagnosis	Secondary Diagnosis
	295.65					
	First-Listed Procedure	Secondary Procedure	Secondary Procedure	Secondary Procedure	Secondary Procedure	Secondary Procedure
	99212	90862				

The provider's diagnosis includes the phrase "in remission" in addition to the term *chronic* to describe the patient's disorder, which means that codes 295.72 and 295.75 are assigned.

This provider is a psychiatrist, which is a medical doctor who reports appropriate level E/M codes for office visits. (If psychotherapy had been provided during the encounter in addition to or instead of an E/M service, the physician would also report an appropriate medicine code, such as code 90805.)

The statement in the notes "This is a 78-year-old white male veteran who is seen for his regular appointment" indicates that this is an established patient. The levels of history and exam are problem focused, and medical decision making is straightforward.

321

POCase004	First-Listed Diagnosis	Secondary Diagnosis	Secondary Diagnosis	Secondary Diagnosis	Secondary Diagnosis	Secondary Diagnosis
	312.00	555.9				
	First-Listed Procedure	Secondary Procedure	Secondary Procedure	Secondary Procedure	Secondary Procedure	Secondary Procedure
	90806					

Do not assign ICD code E932.0 (Adrenal cortical steroids causing adverse effect in therapeutic use) because "Possible reaction to Prednisone" is a qualified diagnosis that is not reported for outpatient care.

Do not assign a CPT E/M code because the psychiatrist provided psychotherapy only.

POCase005	First-Listed Diagnosis	Secondary Diagnosis	Secondary Diagnosis	Secondary Diagnosis	Secondary Diagnosis	Secondary Diagnosis
	311					
	First-Listed Procedure	Secondary Procedure	Secondary Procedure	Secondary Procedure	Secondary Procedure	Secondary Procedure
	99212	90862				

Do not assign code 780.79 (Other malaise and fatigue) for tiredness or 780.95 (Other excessive crying) for tearfulness because they are symptoms of depression (311).

Do not assign ICD code 256.31 (Premature, or early, menopause) because the term *probable* indicates that this is a qualified diagnosis, which is not assigned a code for outpatient care.

The phrase "Mrs. Bronte was seen for recheck" indicates that this is an established patient. The levels of history and exam are problem focused, and medical decision making is straightforward.

NOTE: Do not report a code for telephone services because the patient was seen by the provider in the office for a related E/M service within the previous seven days.

POCase006	First-Listed Diagnosis	Secondary Diagnosis	Secondary Diagnosis	Secondary Diagnosis	Secondary Diagnosis	Secondary Diagnosis
	300.4	414.00	437.9	530.81	272.4	
	First-Listed Procedure	Secondary Procedure	Secondary Procedure	Secondary Procedure	Secondary Procedure	Secondary Procedure
	99213					

This patient does not have a current primary care provider, who would typically monitor his hyperlipidemia, etc. The psychiatrist documents that his practice's office manager will work with the patient to identify a new primary care provider. In the meantime, his practice will treat all of the patient's problems. Thus, ICD codes for each condition documented in the case are assigned.

The statement "Mr. Hall is an 80-year-old white male who was last seen in June of this year for the above problems" indicates that he is an established patient. The levels of history and exam are expanded problem focused, and medical decision making is straightforward.

POCase007	First-Listed Diagnosis	Secondary Diagnosis	Secondary Diagnosis	Secondary Diagnosis	Secondary Diagnosis	Secondary Diagnosis
	781.2	721.0	356.9			
	First-Listed Procedure	Secondary Procedure	Secondary Procedure	Secondary Procedure	Secondary Procedure	Secondary Procedure
	99212					

The phrase "Patient returns for recheck" indicates an established patient. The level of history and exam are problem focused, and medical decision making is moderate complexity.

POCase008	First-Listed Diagnosis	Secondary Diagnosis	Secondary Diagnosis	Secondary Diagnosis	Secondary Diagnosis	Secondary Diagnosis
	355.8					
	First-Listed Procedure	Secondary Procedure	Secondary Procedure	Secondary Procedure	Secondary Procedure	Secondary Procedure
	99212					

To locate ICD code 355.8, go to main term *Neuropathy, neuropathic* and follow the instruction that says "*see also* Disorder, nerve." Then go to main term *Disorder* and subterm *lower limb* to locate code 355.8.

Do not assign ICD code E939.0 as a secondary diagnosis. The statement "symptomatic response to prescribed amitriptyline" in the assessment portion of the SOAP note is not documenting an adverse reaction to medication case. The patient was prescribed the medication (amitriptyline), and the physician documents that the patient's condition (paresthesias) has improved as a result of taking the medication.

Do not assign ICD code 782.0 (Disturbance of skin sensation) because paresthesias are symptoms of the patient's established diagnosis, distal sensorimotor neuropathy.

The phrase as "per previous visit" indicates an established patient. The level of history and exam are problem focused, and medical decision making is straightforward.

POCase009	First-Listed Diagnosis	Secondary Diagnosis	Secondary Diagnosis	Secondary Diagnosis	Secondary Diagnosis	Secondary Diagnosis
	333.1	401.9	434.91			
	First-Listed Procedure	Secondary Procedure	Secondary Procedure	Secondary Procedure	Secondary Procedure	Secondary Procedure
	99212					

Hypertensive vascular disease is coded as hypertension. In the ICD-9-CM Index to Diseases, go to main term *Disease*, subterm *vascular*, and second qualifier *hypertensive* to locate the instruction to "*see* Hypertension."

To locate code 434.91, go to main term *Infarct, infarction* and subterm *cortical* in the ICD-9-CM Index to Diseases.

The phrase "upon recheck" indicates an established patient. The level of history is expanded problem focused, level of exam is problem focused, and medical decision making is moderate.

POCase010	First-Listed Diagnosis	Secondary Diagnosis	Secondary Diagnosis	Secondary Diagnosis	Secondary Diagnosis	Secondary Diagnosis
	110.1	701.1	260.61	357.2		
	First-Listed Procedure	Secondary Procedure	Secondary Procedure	Secondary Procedure	Secondary Procedure	Secondary Procedure
	11721	11056-59				

Report modifier -51 with 11056 to indicate that multiple procedures were performed during this office visit. (The payer will reimburse code 11721 at 100 percent and code 11056-51 at 50 percent.) If modifier -51 is not added to multiple procedure code(s) when the claim is submitted, the payer will reject the claim. The provider will not receive reimbursement until a corrected claim is submitted.

According to Ingenix's Encoder Pro Expert software, directional modifiers are not added to CPT code 11721 or 11056 (e.g., T7 and T8). (After entering a CPT code in Encoder Pro Expert, click the M button on the toolbar to determine which modifiers can be added to the code.) Codes 11721 and 11056 are classified in the CPT Surgery section, Integumentary System subsection; the integumentary system (skin) does not contain paired organs or anatomic sites, although surgery is performed on the skin of a paired anatomic site (e.g., foot).

Do not assign a CPT E/M code because evaluation and management services were not provided.

Workbook Appendix D: Hospital Inpatient Coding Cases

IPCASES ANSWER KEY

IPCase001	Admission Diagnosis	Principal Diagnosis	Secondary Diagnosis	Secondary Diagnosis	Secondary Diagnosis
	780.60	590.10	041.4	276.51	
	Principal Procedure	Secondary Procedure	Secondary Procedure	Secondary Procedure	Secondary Procedure

MS-DRG: 690 (Kidney and urinary tract infections w/o MCC)

Do not report code 305.x for tobacco abuse because it was not medically managed (e.g., treatment or patient counseling).
   Ancillary tests (e.g., IVP, EKG, and chest x-ray) are not usually coded for inpatient cases because the ICD-9-CM codes do not impact DRG grouping. However, your instructor (or the facility at which you become employed) may require you to assign such codes.

IPCase002	Admission Diagnosis	Principal Diagnosis	Secondary Diagnosis	Secondary Diagnosis	Secondary Diagnosis
	366.9	366.9	496	V13.59	
	Principal Procedure	Secondary Procedure	Secondary Procedure	Secondary Procedure	Secondary Procedure
	13.59	13.71			

MS-DRG: 117 (Intraocular procedures w/o CC/MCC)

Do not assign 13.41 for this case because there is no documentation of *phacoemulsification* technique, which is "a method of emulsifying and aspirating a cataract with a low frequency ultrasonic needle." (Stedman's Medical Dictionary) In this case, the patient underwent extracapsular cataract extraction (13.59) with implantation of a lens (13.71). Code V13.59 is assigned based on review of the chest x-ray, which states "old compression fracture of the lower thoracic spine."

IPCase003	Admission Diagnosis	Principal Diagnosis	Secondary Diagnosis	Secondary Diagnosis	Secondary Diagnosis
	521.00	521.00	525.8	428.0	287.30
			414.01	303.93	571.5
	Principal Procedure	Secondary Procedure	Secondary Procedure	Secondary Procedure	Secondary Procedure
	23.19	24.5			

MS-DRG: 168 (Mouth procedures w/o CC/MCC)

Sequence 428.0 in the top five secondary diagnoses, below the principal diagnosis, because it is a comorbidity that impacts the DRG assignment. Under MS-DRGs, code 428.0 is not considered a comorbidity, which means that it does not impact the MS-DRG assignment (or payment). The "unspecified" fifth-digit 0 is added to code 303.9 because documentation in the patient record does not indicate whether the condition is continuous, episodic, or in remission.
   Do not assign ICD-9-CM diagnosis codes for ingrown toenail or abscess (or ICD-9-CM procedure codes for treatment of the conditions); that surgery was performed prior to inpatient admission. Postsurgical care is provided during this inpatient admission and is included in the global period.

325

IPCase004	Admission Diagnosis	Principal Diagnosis	Secondary Diagnosis	Secondary Diagnosis	Secondary Diagnosis
	332.0	276.8	332.0	276.51	
	Principal Procedure	Secondary Procedure	Secondary Procedure	Secondary Procedure	Secondary Procedure

MS-DRG: 641 (Nutritional and miscellaneous metabolic disorders w/o MCC)

IPCase005	Admission Diagnosis	Principal Diagnosis	Secondary Diagnosis	Secondary Diagnosis	Secondary Diagnosis
	303.00	303.90	303.90	V66.4	
	Principal Procedure	Secondary Procedure	Secondary Procedure	Secondary Procedure	Secondary Procedure

MS-DRG: 897 (Alcohol/drug abuse or dependence w/o rehabilitation therapy w/o MCC)

IPCase006	Admission Diagnosis	Principal Diagnosis	Secondary Diagnosis	Secondary Diagnosis	Secondary Diagnosis
	486	482.83	414.01		
	Principal Procedure	Secondary Procedure	Secondary Procedure	Secondary Procedure	Secondary Procedure

MS-DRG: 179 (Respiratory infections and inflammations w/o CC/MCC)

IPCase007	Admission Diagnosis	Principal Diagnosis	Secondary Diagnosis	Secondary Diagnosis	Secondary Diagnosis
	332.0	332.0			
	Principal Procedure	Secondary Procedure	Secondary Procedure	Secondary Procedure	Secondary Procedure

MS-DRG: 057 (Degenerative nervous system disorders w/o MCC)

IPCase008	Admission Diagnosis	Principal Diagnosis	Secondary Diagnosis	Secondary Diagnosis	Secondary Diagnosis
	998.59	998.59	682.2	041.4	112.0
			E878.6	112.0	V10.05
	Principal Procedure	Secondary Procedure	Secondary Procedure	Secondary Procedure	Secondary Procedure
	86.04	97.83			

MS-DRG: 863 (Postoperative and post-traumatic infections w/o MCC)

Assign code 97.83 for removal of staples, as documented in progress note dated 11-18. (The patient was admitted due to infection of surgical wound, but surgical treatment was performed during a previous admission. The staples were also removed during this admission, which means that a code is assigned for staple removal.)

IPCase009	Admission Diagnosis	Principal Diagnosis	Secondary Diagnosis	Secondary Diagnosis	Secondary Diagnosis
	780.39	780.2	780.39	305.1	
	Principal Procedure	Secondary Procedure	Secondary Procedure	Secondary Procedure	Secondary Procedure
	MS-DRG: 312 (Syncope and collapse)				

You might be tempted to assign code 460 for the treatment of the patient's worsening cold. Note that treatment was Tylenol only and that no documentation indicates that the patient's having a cold impacted treatment of the principal diagnosis. Therefore, don't assign code 460.

IPCase010	Admission Diagnosis	Principal Diagnosis	Secondary Diagnosis	Secondary Diagnosis	Secondary Diagnosis
	466.19	466.19	V13.7		
	Principal Procedure	Secondary Procedure	Secondary Procedure	Secondary Procedure	Secondary Procedure
	93.94				
	MS-DRG: 203 (Bronchitis and asthma w/o CC/MCC)				

Answer Key to Workbook Appendix E: Mock Certified Professional Coder (CPC) Certification Examination

1. a	39. d	77. c	115. a
2. b	40. c	78. b	116. c
3. c	41. c	79. b	117. c
4. a	42. b	80. b	118. a
5. d	43. a	81. b	119. a
6. d	44. a	82. a	120. c
7. c	45. d	83. d	121. b
8. a	46. b	84. c	122. b
9. d	47. b	85. c	123. a
10. c	48. c	86. a	124. c
11. d	49. c	87. d	125. b
12. d	50. d	88. a	126. d
13. d	51. c	89. a	127. a
14. b	52. d	90. c	128. b
15. a	53. d	91. c	129. d
16. a	54. c	92. d	130. c
17. b	55. a	93. a	131. b
18. b	56. a	94. a	132. a
19. c	57. c	95. b	133. b
20. d	58. a	96. d	134. a
21. d	59. c	97. b	135. d
22. b	60. c	98. d	136. c
23. d	61. b	99. b	137. b
24. c	62. c	100. b	138. a
25. b	63. a	101. c	139. b
26. b	64. b	102. a	140. b
27. b	65. b	103. a	141. b
28. c	66. c	104. c	142. d
29. d	67. a	105. c	143. b
30. c	68. d	106. b	144. a
31. a	69. d	107. a	145. b
32. b	70. c	108. a	146. b
33. c	71. c	109. b	147. a
34. b	72. a	110. d	148. b
35. b	73. b	111. c	149. b
36. d	74. c	112. b	150. c
37. a, b	75. a	113. c	
38. a	76. c	114. b	

SECTION VII

Answer Key to Workbook Appendix F: Mock Certified Coding Specialist-Physician (CCS-P) Certification Examination

1. b

Note:

HCPCS (CPT and HCPCS level II) and ICD-9-CM are used to completely code this case. ICD-9-CM is used to code the diagnosis, and CPT (level I of HCPCS) is used to code the procedure.

2. d   4. b   5. a
3. a

Note:

The information associated with this question are data elements collected by hospital emergency departments for the Data Elements for Emergency Systems (DEEDS) data set.

6. d   8. b   10. d
7. d   9. a

Note:

CMS's official ICD-9-CM coding guidelines state that when a patient presents for scheduled chemotherapy, a code from category V58 is reported as the first-listed diagnosis code, followed by the cancer code. Code V10.11 is not reported when the patient is undergoing active treatment for a diagnosis such as lung cancer.

11. c   16. c   21. c
12. a   17. b   22. c
13. d   18. a   23. b
14. c   19. c
15. a   20. b

Note:

Review the operative report to locate the depth of the abscess, such as documentation that the surgeon penetrated the fascia. (The fascia is the layer of tissue that connects muscle to skin.) If the fascia is penetrated, determine how far (e.g., muscle, or muscle and bone) and locate the appropriate code in the Musculoskeletal subsection of CPT Surgery. If the surgeon did not penetrate the fascia, report a code from the Integumentary subsection of CPT Surgery instead.

24. a   25. b

Note:

ICD-9-CM contains E codes, which are assigned for mechanism of injury data.

26. a   29. d   32. b
27. d   30. c   33. d
28. c   31. c

> **Note:**
>
> Per the 1995 guidelines, a level 5 E/M code would be reported based on the presenting nature of this patient and the severe life-threatening femoral artery injury. Also, the patient is unable to provide his or her own medical history due to the documented fact that he or she is in and out of consciousness.

34. c

> **Note:**
>
> The physician documented range of motion (ROM) and neurological reflexes. The physician also documented the condition of the patient's skin for the areas of the patient's complaint. This would be an expanded problem focus due to the neurological component and the Integumentary component that is documented.

35. d   36. c

> **Note:**
>
> An open tube bronchoscopy is used to remove foreign objects from the bronchial area.

37. c   38. c   39. a

> **Note:**
>
> No CPT modifier is added, the nose/nares is not a paired organ; therefore, it would be incorrect to assign a modifier -50 to the code for this procedure.

40. a   43. b   46. b
41. a   44. c   47. a
42. d   45. c   48. d

> **Note:**
>
> RAC, or Recovery Audit Contractor, is a program implemented in 2009 under the MMA Act of 2003. CoP is the abbreviation for conditions of participation, NCCI is the abbreviation for National Correct Coding Initiative, and POA is the abbreviation for present on admission. POA is part of the MS-DRG system, which is focused on inpatient services. NCCI provides information on CPT codes to prevent the practice of unbundling. RAC is the most recent of Medicare's initiatives and is focused particularly on overpayments and underpayments.

49. b   52. d   55. c
50. c   53. a   56. c
51. b   54. a

> **Note:**
>
> *Category III codes are temporary codes for emerging technology*

57. c

> **Note:**
>
> *Appendix A of CPT lists level I modifiers. Also in this appendix is a listed of modifiers that are approved for use in ASU outpatient centers. These include modifiers -25, -27, -50, -52, -58, -59, -73, -74, -76, -77, -78, -79, and -91.*

58. b

> **Note:**
>
> *Appendix B contains a summary of additions, deletions, and revisions for the current CPT coding manual.*

59. a   60. b

> **Note:**
>
> *Appendix I contains the genetic testing modifiers that are alphabetic or alphanumeric in format and can be added to both CPT and HCPCS level codes.*